NAT MORRIS

THE CANCER
BLACKOUT

Exposing the official blacklisting of
beneficial cancer research,
treatment and prevention.

". . . there is no disease whose prime cause is better
known. That the prevention of cancer will come there
is no doubt. But how long prevention will be avoided
depends on how long the prophets of agnosticism will
succeed in inhibiting the application of scientific
knowledge in cancer."

Otto Warburg

THE CANCER BLACKOUT

by NAT MORRIS

This printing of THE CANCER BLACKOUT, reflects the many rapid changes in cancerology of the last few years, probably exceeding those of the last century.

To understand cancer, the author writes, it must be considered in its entirety, not only as a disease that has often been mercilessly exploited, but also as a moral cause, as a scientific problem, and a battleground for bitter professional conflicts. How and why, the all powerful professional cliques and organizations have foisted their "treatments of choice" upon the public is realistically exposed.

THE CANCER BLACKOUT reveals many new developments, heralding a new phase in cancer treatment, utilizing the achievements of independent workers and vindicating the heroic struggles of Koch, Ivy, Coffey and Humber, and others whose work is described.

4.50

THE CANCER BLACKOUT

Exposing the official blacklisting of
beneficial cancer research,
treatment and prevention.

by
Nat Morris

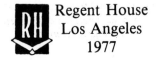
Regent House
Los Angeles
1977

Dedicated to the Memory of the late

Professor Otto Warburg, Nobel Laureate in Medicine, 1931 and 1944. Late Director of the Max Planck Institute for Cell Physiology, Berlin-Dahlem.

"But nobody today can say that one does not know what cancer and its prime cause is. On the contrary, there is no disease whose prime cause is better known, so that today ignorance is no longer an excuse that one cannot do more about prevention. That the prevention of cancer will come there is no doubt, for man wishes to survive. But how long prevention will be avoided depends on how long the prophets of agnosticism will succeed in inhibiting the application of scientific knowledge in the cancer field. In the meantime, millions of men must die unnessarily."

The Prime Cause and Prevention of Cancer

Library of Congress Catalog Card Number 59-7607
International Standard Book Number 911238-61-1
Printed in the United States of America

FOREWORD

In the last five years, more dramatic changes have taken place in cancerology than in the preceeding century. Probably the most significant event is the appalling increase in cancer and its alarming incidence in the very young; now it strikes infants.

In order to understand cancer in its entirety, not only as a disease, but also as a scientific and medical problem, a moral cause against the exploitation of its victims and a source of bitter professional feuds and conflicts, the full gamut of the history of cancer should be reviewed. To reveal all the facets of cancer is the purpose of this study.

By reviewing the past, the tactics of today's powerful professional cliques and organizations dictating "the treatments of choice," can be understood. The Guy-Gataker feud of 1764 was repeated in most of its features in the Krebiozen controversy almost two centuries later. Mr. Gataker, surgeon to His Majesty George III, was not terribly concerned about the danger or ineffectiveness of the "treatments of choice" of that day Mr. Guy warned about, namely hemlock, nightshade, "Cow's dung boiled in milk," warm sea sand, and suchlike, but did rise up against Mr. Guy in anger and hate when he tried to prove the efficacy of his private cancer therapy.

Likewise, the American Medical Association was indifferent to the hazards of reckless irradiation applied to children in the sixties, despite the warnings published in their own journals, now believed to be the cause of cancer erupting in adults exposed to

Xrays in their childhood. At that time, the AMA was too busy fighting the unproven hazards of Krebiozen, to heed their own warnings about radiation.

Is it possible that today's cancer establishmentarians are like Mr. Gataker of 1764 whose cancer fatalities among his royal clientele were so high that he feared the royal wrath if it became known at something better than his treatment was available? If some lowly physician like Guy could discover an effective cancer remedy, how would Gataker's reputation fare at court? Did he attack Guy so viciously to save his own reputation? Was Gataker's motive for discrediting Mr. Guy any different than the American Medical Association's for ruining Professor Ivy?

Nevertheless, the American Cancer Society, the American Medical Association and similar prestigious organizations have performed one important service to the public which has had some interesting repercussions, namely identifying smoking as a cause of lung cancer. Cigarette advertising banned from television and printed advertising, has called attention to other environmental carcinogens, such as air pollution, food preservatives, food substitutes and colorings and hormonal stimulation in meat production. The imminent blacklisting of Red Dye No. 2 and saccharine by the Food and Drug Administration is a logical consequence of associating lung cancer with cigarette consumption.

It was a hard, tough fight to restrict the advertising of the tobacco interests and warn the public on the hazards of smoking, yet the cigarette business still booms. "Coffin nails" are still bought heavily; millions of smokers fully informed on the dangers of their habit, still puff away, willing to risk cancer for the sake of their addiction. Many others are unconvinced and refuse to believe that smoking can result in cancer of the lung.

Even some physicians are still not convinced by the Surgeon General on the hazards of smoking. There is a story current that a psychiatrist testing the sanity of a patient applying for release from a mental institution, asked him why he had quit smoking.

"Because the Surgeon General says it is dangerous," the patient replied.

On that ground, the psychiatrist questioned his sanity and advised against his discharge.

The current interest in diet has also had an important bearing in cancer. Hundreds and hundreds of books are available on the proper selection and preparation of foods and the importance of diet to prevent disease and attain good health. According to Dr. Gerson, a detoxifying diet alone can cure cancer. Almost all the therapies described in this book, stress proper nutrition as an adjunct. It is also preventative. At today's exorbitant costs of medical care, drugs and hospitalization, it is ruinous to become sick even with health insurance or Medicare. Therefore diet has become very important to a person's well being.

Once medical physicians were notoriously indifferent about diet; they were not taught the subject in medical schools, or at best, very briefly. Now they are becoming diet conscious and prescribe such vitamins they ridiculed in the past as Vitamin E. The cholesterol scare has also had its benefits since foods restricted because of their cholesterol forming potentials also may have some carcinogenetic ingredients.

This is interesting progress. In the history of blacklisting by the medical profession, anyone concerned with the quality of the nutriments processed commercially was instantly labeled a "food faddist" or a "food fakir." That sort of derision is no longer possible. Our daily newspapers feature so much material on diet, food qualities and the proper preparation and selection of foods that the medical profession refrains from such derision. There has indeed been progress.

The change in status of independents in cancer work in less than two decades can be gauged from the chapter on "California's Cancer Hearings." At that time, (1959) my testimony was that independent cancer workers were barred from witnessing the tests of their own nostrums by the reigning authorities. When a doctor challenged my statement, and inferred that that was not true, he reversed himself by admitting that it had never been done, because they had "never been asked." I doubt that he could ever get away with so asinine a statement today.

The brutal treatment of Doctor Ivy, a man of magnificent integrity, courage and competence, after he testified in those hearings provides an insight into the character of his enemies and their diabolical tricks. Prior to his work with Krebiozen, Professor Ivy was internationally known and respected, author of hundreds of scientific papers and high in the councils of the organizations who so swiftly turned upon him. As did Mr. Gataker, when they were refused the purchase of Krebiozen, the stream of their invective and defamation was immediately loosed.

The California Hearings of 1959 eventually led to the passage of the Weinberger bill, used to bludgeon proponents of Laetrile and other non-toxic cancer remedies. The current legalization of non-toxic remedies in various states, now numbering twelve, with passage imminent in California and other states, repeals such infamous legislation like the Weinberger bill. Each state that now permits physicians to administer remedies of their own choice providing they are non-toxic, challenges the authority of the Food and Drug Administration to blacklist such nostrums.

Every such bill enacted is a new star in the flag

of freedom of choice in medical treatment; every such bill vindicates the work and struggles of Ivy, Koch, Gerson, Coffey, Humber and other independent workers discussed herein. Every such bill that passes now tactly recognizes that the prime causes of cancer are nutritional deficiencies and environmental carcinogens.

Nat Morris
Los Angeles, California

THE

ANSWER

OF

RICHARD GUY,

Surgeon, in *Mark-lane*,

To certain invidious Falfhoods and Reflections
upon his Method of curing

CANCERS WITHOUT CUTTING,

Lately publifhed in an INTRODUCTION to the
ESSAYS, &c. of

THOMAS GATAKER,

Surgeon Extraordinary to His M efty, &c. &c.

Proper for the Perufal of thofe, who are
in any Degree, afflicte with *Cancers*.

LONDON:

Printed for *R. Willock*, in *Cornhill*; *W. Brifto v*, in *St. Paul's Church-Yard*; and all other Bookfellers in London and *Weft-minfter*. M,DCC,LXIV.

Title Page of Richard Guy's answer to Thomas Gataker.
(Courtesy Northwestern University Medical Library)

CONTENTS

ILLUSTRATIONS

CHAPTER 1

California's Cancer Hearings

D URING the preparation of this book, I was presented with an excellent opportunity not only to witness an inquiry into cancer treatments, but also to participate in it. The occasion was the hearings of the California State Senate's Interim Committee, held in San Francisco, May 6 to 8, 1958. This committee was formed to hear further testimony with a view toward modifying the defeated Weinberger bill, a measure to set up a commission empowered to validate methods of treating cancer and to define the permissible spheres in the treatment of cancer by nonmedically affiliated physicians. A letter to Mr. H. Connolly, Jr., legal counsel for the committee, had resulted in an invitation to testify, on the strength of my statement that I had worth-while material to present.

The original Weinberger bill had been defeated, but its proponents had refused to let it die. This bill is highly important to every citizen, not only in California but in the entire United States, for it may augur a revolutionary attempt to dictate the trends of events in the treatment of cancer and eventually of all other diseases. Not only the life and health of everyone may be involved, but the professional destinies of thousands of practitioners and investigators are also in the balance. When certain approaches to the treatment of a disease are authorized and all others become illegal, every mode of treatment and every avenue of investigation will be narrowly restricted.

The Weinberger bill was sponsored by the American Cancer Society and was introduced in the California legislature on January 21, 1957. Its intent purportedly was to protect the public by illegalizing dangerous and worthless modes of cancer treatment and recognizing only the treatments "of choice," currently surgery, Xray, irradiation and a few chemotherapies. The recommendations of the American Medical Association, the National Cancer Institute, the American Cancer Society, the Sloan-Kettering Institute and similar official bodies would probably determine the sanctioning of cancer therapies.

Opponents of the measure have charged that the bill constituted a means whereby the American Medical Association and its affiliates could extend the same control over practitioners of other schools that it maintains over medical physicians. The AMA exercises its control over the profession by setting up regulations for medical practice which it administers through its various councils. Complaints against the conduct of physicians are heard before an AMA council which for all practical purposes is a court of law.

A physician found guilty of unethical practices is dropped from membership in the AMA. That usually means death to his professional standing, not only because of the disgrace, but because he may no longer send his patients to any hospital affiliated with the American Medical Association. One ground for dismissal from membership is the use of a remedy not approved by the AMA's Council on Pharmacy.

This punishment has been invoked on physicians who have prescribed Glyoxylide, the cancer remedy originated by Dr. William F. Koch which has been the nucleus of a bitter feud since 1919. Krebiozen, the serum sponsored by Dr. Andrew C. Ivy, is also on the blacklist, and although it may be used for experimental purposes, even that use has been fraught with serious hazards to a physician's professional standing. Later chapters will discuss these drugs more fully.

Another serious infraction of American Medical Association rules is the publication, without official permission, of announcements or discussions of remedies in the lay press. The AMA's authority to punish and ostracize its members is exercised legally. A physician who wishes to seek redress for any disciplinary action taken against him can take his case to the civil courts only after he has exhausted every possibility of redress from the American Medical Association itself. There is no instance in which a physician has been successful in such a lawsuit.

One reason for the defeat of the Weinberger bill was the charge of nonmedically trained practitioners that the commission proposed in the bill would be dominated by the AMA. Consequently, they contended, "unorthodox" approaches to cancer, and eventually to all other diseases, would be banned and nonmedical doctors would be deprived of a means of livelihood. In order to hear these charges and secure further data on cancer therapy, the Senate Interim Committee conducted hearings in Los Angeles in the fall of 1957. The San Francisco hearings were called on May 6, 1958, for the same purpose.

The first witness to appear was Glen S. Harman, M.D., a Fellow of the American College of Surgeons, past president of his local surgical society and chief surgeon at the hospital with which he is affiliated. Despite these impressive qualifications, Doctor Harman, who had a folksy and diffident manner, disclaimed any standing as a specialist and modestly described himself as a general practitioner.

Doctor Harman delivered a rather drawn-out, elementary lecture on the diagnosis, pathology and treatment of cancer, illustrated by histological slides of both normal and cancerous tissue. He displayed several diagnostic instruments and explained their use in snipping off tissue for biopsy. He stated that in the most up-to-date practice of surgery, a pathologist is in attendance during an exploratory operation to examine quickly specimen tissue taken from the patient. The pathologist presumably determines on the spot whether a simple operation or radical surgery for extensive cancer involvement should be performed.

Doctor Harman described various types of cancers, as well as the complications arising because of the site and degree of malignancy. In repeating the showing of one slide, he referred to it as again illustrating "our dear friend, the polyps." He also mentioned these "dear friends" as the cause of a case of acute bowel obstruction which he had himself relieved by prompt and effective surgery.

After Doctor Harman's lengthy exposition, the committee chairman asked if there is any truth in the accusation that surgery and radiation treatment aggrevated and spread cancer. In reply, Doctor Harman mentioned the presence of the pathologist in doubtful cases to determine on the spot the extent of cancer involvement and the extent of the operation. This was hardly an answer to the question; nevertheless it was accepted.

"What is the treatment of choice in cancer?" Doctor Harman was asked. He replied that surgery and radiation are the best "at present."

"Are they close to finding a cancer cure?" was another query. Doctor Harman predicted that a cure would be found some day and admitted that surgery is not the ideal treatment for cancer, but only the best available. The ideal remedy might be a serum, he said, capable of creating an immunity to cancer. To the best of his knowledge, no such serum was available.

Among his observations was one that a well-trained physician beginning his practice should be capable of diagnosing cancer.

Another interesting question was whether a cancer might disappear spontaneously, without treatment. Doctor Harman replied that in treating cancer "anything is possible and anything could happen." He stated that purely palliative surgery performed on a patient believed doomed to die was sometimes followed by an unexpected recovery.

To summarize the testimony of Doctor Harman: It covered practically every aspect of the cancer question and directly or indirectly touched upon the most controversial points. It presented the official viewpoint— the recognized stand of the American College of Surgeons and affiliated organizations—and the presentation was practiced and thoroughly memorized. No doubt it was the gist of what Doctor Harman often was called upon to explain to his patients, to their relatives, to his hospital residents and internes and to his colleagues.

The second witness was Fred J. Hart, director of the National Health Federation and the Electronic Medical Foundation, endowed by the late Albert Abrams, at one time a professor of medicine and pathology at Cooper Medical College in San Francisco, and the inventor of various electronic diagnostic instruments. Doctor Abrams died in the early twenties, vilified and discredited by the AMA, despite his high academic and professional standing before he dabbled in medical electronics. He was also the originator of spondylotherapy, which is similar to chiropractic but probably based on more expert knowledge of anatomy and physiology.

There was little in Mr. Hart's testimony that bore directly on the cancer problem. It was more concerned with accusing the AMA of bureaucracy and of hindering freedom of research. Since 1953, a federal injunction has prohibited the Abrams instruments from interstate commerce.

A somewhat comical note was interjected into the hearings when the chairman read a lengthy telegram from an associate of Mr. Hart, accusing the Navy of skulduggery in calling Dr. Joseph Wilson to temporary Navy duty and thus preventing his testimony in behalf of the Drosnes-Lazenby Clinic of Pittsburgh, sponsors of Mucorhicin. To refute this allegation of a plot, Mr. Connolly read some correspondence from Doctor Wilson, written long before the hearings, in which he regretted his inability to appear because of his scheduled duty.

The next witness was to have been Harry M. Hoxsey, probably the most notorious and most colorful figure in the entire history of cancer. When his name was called, there was a dramatic silence. When the call was repeated several times without a response,* the next witness was taken.

That witness was Raymond Kaiser, M.D., of the National Cancer Institute at Bethesda, Maryland. He testified that Congress appropriated $56,000,000 yearly for cancer research, that an additional $30,000,000 is distributed by the American Cancer Society and the

---

* The following day Hoxsey wired the chairman that his attorney had been instructed to explain his absence, but through a misunderstanding had failed to be present at the previous day's hearings. The telegram stated that inasmuch as the single hour alloted for his testimony could not do justice to his testimony which needed at least one full day, he did not think it worthwhile to appear.

Damon Runyon Fund and that this money supports thousands of investigations, 85 per cent of which are done by other than government workers.

An important feature of Doctor Kaiser's testimony was his summary of the established policy of the National Research Council for investigating cancer preparations. Before consenting to investigate a proposed remedy, the Council requires a full disclosure of its chemical formula if an analysis exists; if the chemistry remains unknown, the method of preparation is to be stated.*

Complete laboratory and clinical records are required, together with microscopic confirmation of diagnoses and evidence of the arrest or disappearance of a tumor, the detailed description of any treatment prior to the use of the preparation to be investigated and full data on dosage and laboratory findings prior, during and subsequent to treatment. The National Cancer Institute also reserves the right to determine if the evidence presented justifies further investigation and when such investigation will be made, and to publish its findings when and if it is considered necessary. (Apparently the presence of the discoverer of a cancer remedy during an investigation was not required, at least it was not mentioned.) Doctor Kaiser testified that there had been "no takers" under these conditions.

Under the chemotherapy program of the National Research Council, carried out at the request of govern-

---

* It is well known that biological products cannot always be completely assayed; some constituents remain undetermined for a long time. For example, Krebiozen is derived from the blood of horses which have been inoculated with a tumor incitant and contains some unknown substances. Furthermore, pharmaceutical houses always guard very closely their methods of preparation, and the owners of Krebiozen refused to surrender this information on those grounds. These requisites of the Council therefore appear unreasonable and have become an insurmountable barrier for the investigation of cancer remedies.

ment agencies and pharmaceutical manufacturers, no
agent for the relief of cancer was as yet available to the
medical profession, Doctor Kaiser said. Under questioning, he stated that Krebiozen had never been investigated.*

Senator Richards then brought up the Hoxsey therapy. Reading from prepared material he asked if it
were not true that Hoxsey had submitted 77 case
records for evaluation and that of these cases, 31 had
not lived five years, 25 were submitted without biopsies
and 5 were cases of external cancer. Doctor Kaiser confirmed these figures. The elimination of the remaining
11 cases for a variety of reasons, left not a single proof
of curing cancer by Hoxsey's method.†

Opening the second day of the hearings was Dr. J.
Chester Vorbeck of Ventura, California, a physician in
his late seventies, who prescribes Koch's Glyoxylide.
Upon asked for merely routine information concerning
his background, he spoke at such great length on each
detail that a committee member found it necessary continually to ask him to confine himself to his subject.
The doctor admitted being "prolix" and eventually got
down to the most important feature of his testimony—
a description of how he had been cured of an inoperable
cancer on his scrotum which had grown to the size of
his head. Newspaper accounts transferred the site of
the malignancy to his abdomen, in order not to offend
the sensibilities of readers. One reporter contradicted
Doctor Vorbeck's contention that his cancer had originated from an injury by citing the announcement from

---

* This statement is false, as I attempted to prove in the hearings on
the day following.

---

† The fair investigation of any cancer therapy merely by examining
records is impossible. The patient must be examined at every stage of
treatment and post mortems must be completed. This point will be
elucidated in later pages.

a California convention of physicians that cancer does not originate from injuries.

Because of Doctor Vorbeck's tendency to be "prolix," due to his advanced age, he made a poor witness. Consequently the vital facts about the Koch treatment, the long history of its development, the investigations and controversies it aroused, the clinical results and the scientific background of Koch its discoverer, received a very inadequate presentation at the hearings.

Dr. Andrew C. Ivy then took the stand. He testified incisively and thoroughly on Krebiozen. The doctor opposed the Weinberger bill on the grounds that it could strangle freedom of research. He was emphatic in his denunciation of the faked investigations of Krebiozen (to be more fully discussed later) which had branded the remedy as worthless.

After ninety minutes, lunch recess was at hand. Doctor Ivy was courteously offered more time, part of which I agreed to relinquish from my own. After the recess, the chairman read the telegram from Hoxsey explaining his absence of the day before.

On resuming his testimony, Doctor Ivy made an interesting and startling disclosure—his first public admission that he had privately investigated the Hoxsey Clinic and cancer cure under an agreement that his visit was to be kept secret.

Doctor Ivy's testimony was not particularly flattering to Hoxsey. He attributed Hoxsey's cures to the potassium iodide in the preparation; and while he acknowledged that the Hoxsey method secures results with external cancer, he said that a paste prepared by the University of Wisconsin does the same. Doctor Ivy did suggest, however, that the Hoxsey method deserved further investigation and that a scientific test of it by the "double blind method" ought to be conducted.

I followed on the stand, intending to testify concerning the methods used in the past to evaluate independently discovered cancer remedies. Not one investigation, so far as I had been able to discover, had ever been
conducted in a fair, impartial and scientific manner. I
was prepared to discuss the investigations of Krebiozen;
the Coffey-Humber extract, which originated in San
Francisco and which probably was well known because
of the great amount of publicity it had received in its
day; and Koch's Glyoxylide. Time permitted my pre-
senting only a small fraction of my material; however,
it will be found in later pertinent chapters.

In referring to Doctor Kaiser's testimony, I called
attention to the fact that the conditions of the National
Cancer Institute's investigations did not call for discoverers to be on hand during investigations. Under
the impression that Doctor Ivy was still in the room, I
said that he would bear me out that Krebiozen had
never been tested in his presence. Doctor Ivy, however,
had already left.

Mr. Connolly interrupted me at this point. "I
want to determine the truth of that statement that the
discoverer of a cancer remedy would no be permitted
to witness its investigation. Does anyone here know
whether he would be forbidden to be present?" he asked.

Doctor Kaiser volunteered to clarify that point and
was ushered to a microphone. It was the only instance
during the hearings that two persons of conflicting view-
points confronted each other, face to face.

"The discoverer of a cancer remedy would be permitted to be present during a test," Doctor Kaiser
affirmed.

"But it has never been done," I told him.

He admitted that was so. When asked why, he
answered, "Because we have never been asked."

This highly curious and somewhat puerile admission came from the spokesman of a government institution, supposedly impartial, and the recipient of $56,000,000 a year for cancer research. Doctor Kaiser had also apparently overlooked his testimony of the previous day that there had been "no takers" from independent workers under the conditions imposed by the National Research Council for testing cancer remedies. It is highly possible that these conditions are considered so unfair by proponents of a cancer remedy that they believe it useless to witness any test.

Because Doctor Kaiser had also testified the day before that Krebiozen had never been tested by the National Research Council, I requested permission to read into the record the evidence* which contradicts that testimony and which proves that the National Research

---

* That evidence was the following letter, published in the *Journal of the American Medical Association* of November 24, 1951:

KREBIOZEN
To the Editor:
At the October 12, 1951 meeting of the Committee on Cancer Diagnosis and Therapy, the following opinion regarding "Krebiozen" was formulated:
The Committee on Cancer Diagnosis and Therapy has reviewed available data on the effects of a secret preparation called "Krebiozen" in the treatment of a large number of cases of cancer. The preparation was used as directed in the original publication of Doctors Durovic and Ivy. The Committee finds no evidence of any curative effect and no proof of palliative effect attributable to the "drug" itself.
This opinion is based on examination of (a) the original booklet prepared by the head of the Department of Clinical Science of the University of Illinois in March, 1951 (b) a summary of 63 cases reviewed by the staff of the Committee; and (c) an analysis of 100 cases prepared by a study committee of the American Medical Association, which 100 cases include some of those referred to under (b).

M. C. Winternitz, M.D., Chairman
Division of Medical Sciences
National Research Council
2101 Constitution Avenue
Washington 25, D.C.

Council had accepted without question the secret tests of Krebiozen conducted by the American Medical Association.

Upon my request to read this letter into the record Mr. Connolly suggested a recess. The Chairman, however, hinted broadly that a recess would be unnecessary as my testimony would be soon concluded. In this way, they foiled my attempt to put the letter into the record.

Under these conditions, I testified on how the Coffey-Humber extract had been evaluated solely on an "investigation" which was conducted by one man and which consisted merely of perusing case histories. Whatever the merits or demerits of the remedy, that one appraisal had been final, despite the endorsement of many outstanding physicians and surgeons, despite the careful observance of medical and scientific procedures, and despite the cures claimed of patients considered to be in the disease's terminal stage.

There was no opportunity for me to introduce into the record the Hardin Jones' statistics on cancer,[1] which compared the survival rates of untreated cancer patients with those who had submitted to surgery and irradiation and which showed that those who had refused treatment lived longer on the average.

Nor was there time to get into the record the test conditions for Glyoxylide, the Koch remedy, which had been set up in 1920 through the influence of Mayor Couzens of Detroit. Cancer patients were to be diagnosed and selected by a committee formed by the Wayne County Medical Society and the patients were to be turned over to Doctor Koch for treatment under the committee's observation. Although these conditions were carried out with only one patient, and the test was eventually called off because both Koch and the committee accused each other of failing to adhere to the conditions, it seemed to me as the fairest and most practical method of investigation ever proposed. I had hoped to suggest to the committee that method of evaluating cancer remedies under an impartial authority empowered to adjudicate disputes between rival interests in cancer, but time ran out.

Dr. Cornelius Rhoads, director of the Sloan-Kettering Institute for Cancer Research, then took the stand, pretending at first to be timid about testifying as an expert because of Doctor Ivy's observation on the notorious unrealiability of so-called "expert" opinions. After this attempt at humor, Doctor Rhoads read from a prepared statement.

Never a day passes, he said, that the Institute is not offered a cancer remedy to test, but there simply is no time to investigate. Among other of his statements were these: Cancer is now being cured in about 40 per cent of cases (whether this included skin cancer, which is regarded as 90 per cent curable, was not clarified); cancer detected early has a greater chance of cure; surgery and irradiation are still the treatments of choice, but some chemotherapeutic methods are proving valuable.

Doctor Rhoads said that there is great unreliability and uncertainty about the diagnosis of cancer and that diagnoses submitted to the Sloan-Kettering Institute from all over the United States are often questioned. Only the day before, however, Doctor Harman had testified that a physician just entering practice should be able to diagnose cancer correctly.

To summarize, Doctor Rhoads got into the record the well known and standardized data, disseminated by the American Cancer Society and similar organizations, which are so familiar they need little further repetition.

The third and last day of the hearings was confined to the testimony of those in agreement with that view-point. Consequently they had the "last word." First on the stand was Dr. Howard Bierman, director of the City of Hope of Los Angeles, a charitable cancer hospital.

Upon being questioned about quack treatments, he related the case of a boy with leukemia, treated first by a highly qualified physician who had secured an excel-lent remission of symptoms, although the life expectancy of leukemia patients is only one or two years at most. Despite the best attainable result under the circum-stances, the boy's mother had insisted on trying a quack remedy. But after a few months on that treatment, she had brought the boy to Doctor Bierman in the most advanced and hopeless condition he had ever seen.

After this account, the doctor was asked about the Hoxsey treatment. He then acknowledged that the leukemia case he had described had been given the Hoxsey therapy, thus inferring his extreme condition was due to the pernicious results of quackery. (One newspaper reported that the boy had been treated first by the Hoxsey method and had become hopeless as a result, although according to the testimony, a qualified physician had first treated him for his leukemia which Doctor Bierman had admitted was hopeless from the start. This is a fair sample of the accuracy of the re-porting on the hearings. Except for the San Francisco *Chronicle,* it was highly inept and biased.)

A surgeon from Dallas, Texas, the home of the Hoxsey therapy, testified next. Because of his prox-imity to the Hoxsey Clinic, he felt that he was able to testify to its dangerous and harmful nature. He called Hoxsey's standing offer to post a huge sum of money and to give up his treatment if he could not cure cancer,

pure showmanship and unworthy of serious consideration.

The next two witnesses were Paul Kirk, Ph.D., Professor of Criminalistics at the University of California
and an authority on chemistry and toxicology, and
Arthur Furst, Professor of Pharmacology at Stanford
University. They had both assayed Krebiozen, and
testified that their tests had been made independently
and without each other's knowledge. From samples not
supplied them directly by the Krebiozen Foundation,
both had come to the same conclusion—that Krebiozen
is little different from mineral oil and contains no active
biological substance.*

Dr. L. Henry Garland, Professor of Radiology at
Stanford University School of Medicine, then followed
on the stand. He claimed that radiological treatment
is about 40 per cent curative in cancer. During the
usual questioning, a member of the committee referred
to my statement that the discoverer of a cancer remedy
is forbidden to be present during tests, and asked Doctor
Garland to confirm that was not true, which he did.
He was then asked about the Coffey-Humber extract.

"I was present in this very room [the Supervisor's
Chambers, San Francisco Hall]," he said, "when Doctor
Coffey was granted $200,000. His patients died like
flies, and the extract had no capacity to relieve pain,
as the nurses' charts showed."

Gordon Granger, M.D., Chief, Drugs and Devices
Branch of the Food and Drug Administration, followed
on the stand, to testify chiefly about the Hoxsey treat-

---

* Doctor Ivy was not available for comment; as he was en route to
Chicago at the time. The Durovics bitterly assailed this testimony and
threatened a lawsuit. They announced they would secure chemical
assays, from reliable independent laboratories, which would be highly
scientific and trustworthy and would completely disprove the findings
of Doctors Kirk and Furst.

ment. He spoke at length about the labeling of drugs and said that the presentation of Hoxsey's book, *You Don't Have to Die,* to a patient during treatment could legally be interpreted as false labeling under the provisions of the Pure Food and Drug Act.

The hearings were terminated by the testimony of Howard Hassard, attorney for the California State Medical Association, on the need for protective legislation against cancer quackery.

This constitutes a brief summary of the California "cancer quack" hearings. How fair were the hearings? How deeply into the matter did the committee delve? Are there undisclosed, hidden and suppressed facts about cancer that it refused to consider? Is the disease serious and deadly, or has its virulent nature been highly exaggerated in terms of total population? What are the motives of some of the men and organizations involved in cancer?

In order to answer these questions, it is necessary to review the many controversies in the history of the disease. The reader will learn that every discoverer of a cancer remedy has encountered a "Chinese wall of resistance." The arguments to discredit independent therapies have been the same all through history. The California hearings were but another battle in the cancer war, although on a much greater scale than earlier ones. Yet the strategy, the weapons, the fierceness of the conflict and the issues involved remain much the same. The same arguments reverberate throughout the history of cancer—arguments tinged with emotion, with prejudice and with violent antagonisms.

A number of myths also have been in circulation. The most misleading one is that the discoverer of a cancer cure will be honored, acclaimed and practically deified as a saviour of the human race. The grim, undistorted facts on record should dispel belief in any such myth. Indeed, any proponent of a cure for one of man's most dreaded diseases is far more likely to be dishonored, denounced and crucified, unless he is a fair haired boy of the dominating oligarchy. To understand this fore-boding first, let us consult the pages of history.

From the San Francisco *Chronicle,* May 8, 1958.

By Elmont Waite

Two men who have been prominent for many years in medical science disagreed sharply here yesterday over how best to protect the public from quacks.

Dr. Andrew C. Ivy of the University of Illinois warned against setting up any State agency that would attempt to list medical treatments as good or bad.

Dr. C. P. Rhoads, director of the Sloan-Kettering Institute in New York, and active in cancer research for 31 years, called it "a proper duty to establish such a body to protect the public" against un-proved methods of treatment.

From the San Francisco *Examiner,* May 9, 1958.

By JOHN F. ALLEN

Cancer "cure" pills peddled by Harry M. Hoxsey of Texas are worse than useless; they hasten the death of human and animal victims.

Krebiozen, another supposed anti-cancer chemical, and the source of a bitter controversy raging around the head of Chicago's Dr. Andrew Ivy, is simply "a good grade of mineral oil and nothing else."

These new and startling accusations constituted the sworn testimony of a parade of expert witnesses who appeared here yesterday before a hearing of the State Senate Interim Commitee on Public Health.

CHAPTER 2

The Pattern of Controversy

Turn back the years to one o'clock on the afternoon of January 5, 1764. Two celebrated London surgeons had agreed to meet at that hour at the Smyrna Coffee House in Pall Mall. Their parley is noteworthy in the history of cancer, just as many of the conversations over coffee at the Smyrna, a favorite meeting place of poets, musicians and members of the court, came to be reflected in the literature and history of the British Empire.

Mr. Richard Guy, a member of the corporation of surgeons of London, well known for his treatment of "scirrhous tumours and cancers" without surgery, arrived promptly. Some of Mr. Guy's colleagues entrusted members of their families to his care; others criticized him caustically for abandoning the knife and adopting a cancer remedy purchased from a layman.

Ten minutes late, but apologizing politely for his tardiness, arrived Mr. Thomas Gataker, "Surgeon Extraordinary to His Majesty, to Her Royal Highness, the Princess Dowager of Wales, to Her Majesty's Household and St. George Hospital."

As their coffee was served, the two surgeons began their confidential talk. Their meeting in such surroundings instead of in a more professional setting was itself significant. As they conversed, their tones became sharp and angry. Unable to agree, after about an hour, they parted with decided coolness.

Angry and suspicious, Mr. Guy hailed his waiting carriage and began immediately to scrawl notes of their conversation on the back of an envelope. On arriving at his home, he called for quill and paper and quickly wrote out a more detailed account while the facts were still fresh in his memory. Later he made full use of that transcript.

To understand their quarrel, it is necessary to review the events which brought the surgeons Guy and Gataker together at the Smyrna Coffee House that January day of 1764. In 1759, Mr. Guy had published *An Essay on Scirrhous Tumours and Cancers, to which are Added the Histories of Cases Cured by the Author by Means of Mr. Plunkett's Medicine.* Mr. Guy's purchase of the medicine had led to the sharp disapproval of his colleagues and he had published his tract "to acquaint the Public with the Reason and Manner of my obtaining Acquisition" and to counteract the "invidious reflections" he had suffered.

He confessed that on first becoming apprized of Mr. Plunkett's claim to a cancer cure, he considered it "but a pretense." But on observing that Plunkett was "attended by a number of unhappy objects which appeared incurable with Cancer" who, after only a few weeks of treatment, seemed miraculously cured, he admitted becoming strongly interested and thinking that with his greater professional competence he could greatly improve the remedy.

The Plunkett poultice had been a family secret for over a century. There are many instances in the history of mankind of nostrums, compounded by laymen, with sacred and secret ingredients having a great healing power not always recognized by physicians. Mr. Guy cited from Helmont, a contemporary authority on cancer, who mentioned a man in the Duchy of Juliens "who cured all sorts of Cancer by sprinkling an indolent and mild Powder upon them, and afterwards an incarn-ing Plaister; but the Secret died with him."

In a fascinating literary style, Mr. Guy discoursed on the necessity and reasons for treating cancer without the knife. Because of the excruciating pain, he wrote, "few or no women would submit to have a Breast cut off were they not persuaded of there being no Alterna-tive but that of Death." In those days, it must be re-called, there was neither anesthesia nor aseptics; the surgeon stropped his knife upon his boots. As he oper-ated, he breathed and coughed into the incision, exposed also to the dust in the room and the particles falling from his beard and hair. The patient was strapped to the table and held down by attendants as the knife cut his quivering flesh or a saw hacked off his bones amid fearful shrieks of pain.

The dread of such excruciating agony caused people to permit their disease to progress to advanced stages before consulting a physician. The disease was then un-mistakable because of the stench of rotting flesh and the gruesome forms of the growth. Mr. Guy described cancers which in some instances had eaten away half the face or an entire breast, exposing the bones under-neath. His essay is replete with remarkably sharp and competent observations. For example:

"The site of a Cancer causes different effects in accordance with the function of neighboring parts which are compressed or otherwise injured; if a Scirrhous presses upon a large Artery it will occasion an atrophy, or wasting, if upon the Trunks of the Veins, oedematous and inflammatory Tumors; if upon the Nerves, Numbness and Torpidness."

He also quoted a number of eminent contemporary authorities. One, Van Swieten, had observed "that so long as a *Scirrhous* possesses any part of the body, it is plain there is Reason to be in continuous Dread of something worse succeeding," indicating that the danger of metastases was recognized even in those days.

Wiseman, another contemporary, was quoted as having written: "In treating a *scirrhous* you are not to use Repellents, for they increase the Disorder."

Heiser was also quoted:

"If you apply a repellent or astringent Medicine to a Scirrhous, the Disorder increases wonderfully; insomuch that one month will produce more increase of Pain and Tumor, than a Year without any medicinal Application."

Before describing his own remedy, Mr. Guy mentioned others then in vogue. These included "Mercurials, gentle friction, Fumes of Vinegar, Plaisters composed of the ferulaceous Gum as Galbomen, Amoniacum, etc., Fomentations of emollient and discutient Herbs, Venice-soap dissolved in Milk, fresh Cow's dung boiled in Milk to the consistence of a Poultice, warm Sea-sand, and human fat."

Of all these concoctions Mr. Guy pessimistically wrote: "If those who have tried all the most favored Medicines . . . will be ingenuous, they must certainly own that their success has been but very indifferent."

Keenly aware of the danger of spreading a tumour, he cautioned against continuing with a remedy unless good results were apparent at once. He warned that body parts adjacent to a tumour also could become cancerous when unduly irritated. He also pointed to the danger of failing to extirpate a tumour completely, and cited a breast operation followed by the rapid eruption of a cancerous fungus as big as a man's head, with holes large enough to accommodate a fist. Caustics were then applied to the fungus but the patient soon expired.

Mr. Guy described the successful treatment of a lip cancer which he had dressed with his remedy in the presence of another physician, contrary to his usual secrecy. The cure required less than a month, although he claimed that ten weeks was the usual course for a cure. He supplied names and addresses of patients he had healed, "for the truth of which the Persons herein mentioned, are referred to, for the further Satisfaction of those who desire it." He further attested that in two years he had applied the Plunkett remedy in one hundred cases without failing in "ten instances where I had hopes of succeeding."

In August, 1762, Mr. Guy published "Practical Observations on Cancer," which supplemented his previous essay and expanded his list of successful treatments to 100 cases. He also appraised two other remedies he had tried without success—nightshade and hemlock. The latter had been introduced by Stork, a physician from Vienna, and Mr. Guy affirmed that in 100 cases he had treated at the Manchester Infirmary, hemlock had merely stupified some and brought blindness to others.

Nightshade had been accepted on the strength of a single case related by a foreign Doctor Lambergen. Mr. Gataker had been so favorably impressed (as Mr. Guy reminded him later) that he had published an endorsement. Mr. Guy, however, warned that "its effects were attended with several not only disagreeable, but very alarming symptoms, for which Reason it since seems to be totally disregarded." Mr. Guy concluded his essay with the descriptions of his 100 cancer cures which had attracted Mr. Gataker's interest and had led to the quarrel after the Smyrna Coffee House meeting to negotiate for the use of the Plunkett remedy. After their meeting, Mr. Gataker published reflections on the skill and competence of Mr. Guy and also accused him of losing patients through neglect. He also scoffed at the notion of "cancerous roots," entertained by Mr. Guy.

Guy's verbuttal, published from his notes immediately after the meeting at the Smyrna Coffee House appeared in 1762 as *The Answer of Richard Guy, Surgeon in Mark-Lane, to certain invidious Falsehoods and Reflections upon his Method of curing Cancer without cutting, lately published in an introduction to the Essays of Thomas Gataker, Surgeon to His Majesty, etc.*

In disclosing their conversation, Mr. Guy wrote that Mr. Gataker immediately tried to secure his formula, suggesting that it be released as a "Public Service." Mr. Guy replied that he could not afford to "lay it open without a Consideration," as he himself had acquired it only after considerable expense and effort and he owed it to his family to secure reimbursement.

As their conversation proceeded, Mr. Guy wrote, he perceived that Mr. Gataker's real interest was not in doing the public a service but only in trying "to sift something" out. A mutual antipathy then arose, after which Mr. Guy confessed he gave only "indefinite answers" to Gataker's further inquiries.

Mr. Gataker then mentioned some unfortunate results with the Plunkett medicine. Mr. Guy acknowledged that these sometimes occurred, but offered to produce fifty or more cases of authentic cures. Mr. Gataker declined to review the cures, and Mr. Guy further accused him of assuming a somewhat "supercilious Air" when he was invited to follow the treatment of an entirely new case.

Their talk ended on this note of rejection and antagonism. Although convinced that his colleague had "no intention of doing the Public a Service but to become his Rival," Mr. Guy nevertheless sent a new pa-

tient with a breast tumor to His Majesty's surgeon before commencing treatment. Declining at first to see
her, Gataker finally consented, only to attempt to lure
her into accepting surgery, according to Guy. "That,"
he thundered, "may show your dirty Disposition to
supplant me!"

However, the patient remained loyal and began her
treatment. A friend of the patient who was also well
acquainted with Gataker, then suggested that she see
him again. This suggestion had probably originated
with Gataker, Guy asserted. The patient refused the
suggestion but indicated she would permit Gataker to
examine her again if they should meet at the home of
their mutual friend. They did eventually meet there.
Guy charged that Gataker then evinced no further interest in another examination, although he surely must
have known through the patient's intimate woman
friend that she had been relieved of her tumor.

In an inimitable style, Mr. Guy thundered his indignation, his contempt and his resentment of his high
placed adversary's sly tactics. The following eloquent
passage is not only a magnificent example of his writ-
ings but states the grievances of those discriminated
against, in a classic fashion:

"And if it were the common practice of Physicians and Surgeons to use the same Inveteracy against
each other, as you have showed to me on account of
unavoidable Accidents; I say, if upon such occasion
they were to be continually charged with the want
of skill or Integrity, it would destroy Reputations so
fast, that the patients must be left without Hope,
and the Practitioners without Practice. . . . How
easy it is for a man desirous of injuring the Reputation of another, to suggest things which he cannot
form into a direct Charge or Accusation. You sup-

PRACTICAL OBSERVATIONS

ON

CANCERS

AND

DISORDERS OF THE BREAST,

EXPLAINING THEIR DIFFERENT

APPEARANCES AND EVENTS.

TO WHICH ARE ADDED,

ONE HUNDRED CASES,

SUCCESSFULLY TREATED WITHOUT CUTTING.

By RICHARD GUY, Surgeon,

And Member of the Corporation of SURGEONS
in *London.*

ALSO

Some Remarks on the Effects of HEMLOCK

SHEWING

The Inefficacy of that Medicine in CANCEROUS
COMPLAINTS.

The Whole serving as a SUPPLEMENT to a former
ESSAY on the Subject, by the same AUTHOR,
August 1762.

L O N D O N:

Printed for W. OWEN, near *Temple-Bar*; W. BRISTOW,
in *St. Paul's Church-yard*; and R. WILLOCK, in *Cornhill.*

Title Page of Guy's *Magnum Opus.*
The four excerpts following illustrate his remarkable insight into
the diagnosis, treatment and pathology of cancer. Note especially
his exposition of metastases and of viruses as a cause of cancer
which would credit any modern cancerologist.

CAUTIONS

CANCEROUS COMPLAINTS.

EXPERIENCE sufficiently e-
vinces, that the fatal Consequences
attending Cancers are many Times
the Effects of Inattention, Neglect,
or improper Treatment in the Infant State
of the Disease, some proof of which may
be deduced from the Cases just mentioned.

As the Symptoms usually preceding almost every Cancer of the Breast, or what
may with Propriety be termed incipient
Cancers*, likewise demonstrate how easily
in that State they are remediable by Care
and proper Management; and what Changes
they undergo by Length of Time, even such
as put it beyond the Power of all Art to re-
cover. For Example, when there are manifest Appearances of a diseased Gland in
the Breast enlarging to a considerable Size,
and seeming to have acquired a perfect schirrous State, attended with Pain; if, after having resisted the Endeavours for Resolution,
the Tumour should remain obdurate, the
Safety of the Patient then requires the speedy
Removal

* Vid. the first ten Cases.

JANE Franklin, from *Knightsbridge*, afflicted with a schirrous Gland about the Size of a Walnut, just in the Bend of the Elbow, took the Hemlock for a long Time under the Direction of an experienced Surgeon: She found not the least Benefit from it; the Gland became adherent and immoveable, attended with acute Pains that struck up to the axillary Glands.

The above Cases may shew, that the Hemlock was possessed of no specific Virtue, either toward curing or abating the Progress of Cancers. I think it unnecessary to remonstrate farther upon it, seeing among those Instances it was given under the Directions of very eminent Persons of the Faculty; and where every Advantage that could have been obtained from it might have succeeded; nor does it appear that its Effects are so innocent to the Constitution, as Dr. *Stork* seems to insist upon.

CAU.

WHOEVER reflects, that the Breasts are composed of almost innumerable small Glands, lymphatic and lactiferous Ducts, Blood-vessels, Nerves, Membranes, &c. all of the most delicate Texture, and most exquisite Sensibility, will not wonder at their being more particularly susceptible of morbid Affections, as well from internal as external Causes.

How readily Obstructions may be formed, either from Disease or Accident, in these very minute and complicated *Tubuli*, must be obvious to even the most moderately qualified Physiologist: The Consequence of such Obstructions commonly are small Lumps or Swellings,

But plausible as this Opinion may seem, it is surely very controvertible; for, suppofing such a putrid Contamination of the *Mafs of Blood* really to exift, it is natural to expect, that its Effects would be visible in the Portions of Blood, drawn by Phlebotomy from the unhappy Subjects of this Difeafe; whereas nothing is more true, than that in Perfons labouring under the moft inveterate and moft malignant Circumftances of an ulcerated Cancer, the Blood is, in general, found as firm in its Texture, and as well proportioned with refpect to its Contents, as in thofe who enjoy the moft perfect Health.

May it not therefore be, with more Probability, inferred, that the cancerous Humour is a Virus, *fui Generis*; that it is originally formed in the Glands, and that the lymphatic Veffels are the immediate Inftruments of its Circulation? May it not be reafonably prefumed, that the morbid Matter of an ulcerated Cancer is reabforbed by thofe Veffels, and by them be carried and lodged in the neighbouring Glands, and from thence to thofe more remote? *viz.* from the Breaft to the Axillary, &c. from
the

pose I may possibly have *selected* successful Cases, and fairly stated them at first, and taken advantage of interesting circumstances; I am glad you only *suppose* so, for I should have been sorry to deserve the censure of doing so; though if this had been the Case, I should only have followed the example of some others."

Every feature of the Guy-Gataker cancer controversy can be observed throughout the history of cancer disputes, until this very day. Accusations of attempts to steal a prized, secret formula without payment, followed by contumely derision and character assassination after such attempts were frustrated, recur constantly. Mr. Guy's charges that his rival tried to lure his patient away from him, that his offers to demonstrate cures were ignored and that known instances of cures were deliberately suppressed, occur again and again in the history of cancer therapy. A study of cancer feuds over the centuries, will show that every feature of the quarrel between the two English surgeons of almost two centuries ago, is almost standard and the pattern of controversy is still essentially the same.

CHAPTER 3

Cancer in the 19th Century

IN PAST centuries, cancer was not a prevalent disease. Before the modern era, conditions of life were so hazardous and sanitation so poor that typhoid fever, smallpox, syphilis, tuberculosis and other infectious diseases took huge tolls of human life. Cancer, therefore, had little chance to develop. It is also believed in some quarters that infectious diseases with their attendant fevers provide an immunity against cancer and that the rise of cancer in recent decades can be attributed to the decline in infectious diseases with a correlated decline in the capacity to develop immunity against other diseases.

The problem of cancer was first recognized in 1802 when the Society for Investigating the Nature and Cause of Cancer was organized in London. Although the society was short-lived, its basic approach is still followed by contemporary cancer societies and organizations.

Virchow published his cellular discoveries about a century ago, and the theory of cancer as a disease of the cells was then adopted. Today this theory is being challenged in favor of a biochemical approach which postulates that the changes in the cells reflect only the metabolic influences which cause the disease. But at that time the detailed study of the structure of tumors, the classification of their varieties was in progress. Irritation, injury and infection were then advanced as causes of the disease. The era of research opened with the twentieth century.

The literature on cancer healing was sparse until only recent years. A cancer cure was a closely guarded secret and was regarded as valuable property, judging from a pamphlet published in Rhode Island in 1784. It was written by Hugh Martin, Physician and Surgeon in the American Army, and was titled *A Narrative of a Discovery of a Sovereign Specific for the cure of Cancers with several other improvements made in Medicine with a postscript on a singular case of a stone taken out of the tongue and is now republished with the addition of extraordinary cures performed by Doctor John Newman of Newport, Rhode Island.*

The remedy was probably an escharotic but was not described. In fact, nothing of great significance was disclosed beyond a bold claim of an efficient cancer remedy.

The great English surgeon and teacher, John Abernethy, contributed much to the technique of removing and classifying tumors. At times he was gloomy about the value of surgery and once observed: "I have known a patient to die soon after an operation for removal of a cancer of not great magnitude, merely in consequence of the shock."

Abernethy called attention to the dietary cancer cure of William Lambe, M.D., of London, who in 1809 published a treatise advocating a diet of fruits, vegetables and pure water. Lambe was one of the pioneers in advocating a vegetarian and fruit diet which he eventually extended to the treatment of all diseases.

BLAKE OF NEW YORK

The cancer situation in the United States is reflected in an interesting pamphlet, *Cancers Cured without the*

Use of the Knife, published in 1858 by T. T. Blake, M.D., of New York. The opening paragraph reads:

"Any treatment of disease that claims to be in advance of what is known to the profession however clearly on scientific principles or uniformly commended by its power to heal, is sure to meet with opposition. In the treatment of cancer that is the more to be expected inasmuch as cancer has been the opprobrium of the profession. By physicians, the world over, it has for the most part been regarded as incurable. If this is not so, why the conviction universally pervading the public mind that all ordinary means to arrest it are impotent?"

The author was quite careful to guard the nature of his remedy, a salve or ointment applied externally. The testimonials of patients and the endorsement of physicians, leading citizens, clergymen and others, profuse in their praise, were liberally sprinkled throughout the work.

According to the testimonial of one, Gideon Langdon, the treatment destroyed the life of his cancer in fifty minutes. "The growth was entirely removed and had healed in three weeks," he was quoted as saying. "There was little pain connected with the treatment which also consisted of internal medication to purify the blood." Langdon also commented upon the satisfaction experienced by many fellow patients with their progress and improvement in health under Doctor Blake's regimen.

The doctor gave an interesting description of his method in contrast to surgery, which he believed was unable to cure but offered only "a respite from impending doom." His own procedure, he claimed, was attended with slight or no pain and was administered in from fifteen to sixty minutes, depending on the extent of the growth. Doctor Blake stressed the value of rapid therapeutic action in order to avoid irritation of the skin believing that a cancer must be cured quickly if it is to be cured at all. Thus Dr. Blake's opinion was the same as that of Richard Guy, published a century earlier.

The Blake treatment brought a discharge from the malignancy after a few days, which continued abundantly until the cancer disappeared. Only slight inflammation occurred around the cancerous area, Blake claimed, in contrast to the increasing inflammation and swelling produced by most cancer remedies after the first application. Doctor Blake boasted that his treatment required no confinement but that the patient could go about his affairs; neither was there any danger of "taking cold" during his treatment, nor any weakening or drain upon the system, as the pulse was not even quickened.

Such claims would be considered pure quackery today. The testimonials of many leading citizens, however, made the Blake claims impressive. Blake boasted of complete cures without recurrence, but his description of the remedy indicated merely that it was purely vegetable in nature and that it contained no poison. He also claimed it could remove wens, birthmarks, moles and all sorts of growths.

THE FELL REMEDY

In all probability, Doctor Blake's treatment was identical to one perfected by Dr. J. Weldon Fell, a contemporary and a most remarkable man and physician. Doctor Fell came from an old and distinguished American family and numbered among his forebears and relatives several famous physicians and profess-

ional men. A cousin was reputed to have induced
Abraham Lincoln to go into politics.

Dr. J. Weldon Fell was also one of the original
founders of the New York Academy of Medicine and
a faculty member of the University of New York.
However, a sinister cloud enveloped his career because
of his cancer practice and in the prime of his life, he
emigrated to London to start anew. There he engaged
again in the practice of cancer under very auspicious
circumstances for he was singularly prosperous and
lived very lavishly. His story is one of the most interesting in the history of cancer. [2, 3]

The real reason for his departure from New York
is still a mystery but it is certain that he was under
a professional cloud. According to the sparse evidence
available, Doctor Fell attempted to resign from the
New York Academy of Medicine, but his resignation
was refused. It seemed that he had become associated
with a cancer quack, one Gilbert of New York City,
and this association had aroused the deep animosity
of his colleagues. Ostracism followed and the acceptance of his resignation was continually postponed in
the hope of pinning a charge of quackery upon him
so he could be ignominiously ejected from the academy.

Evidently Doctor Fell had accumulated a sizeable
fortune before he became disgraced. He took his family to Europe and later wrote a friend of renting a
castle for $100 per week, certainly a munificent sum
in those days. He also retained quite a staff of serv-
ants. After opening his office, he was quite successful
even though a Yankee and a foreigner in effete London.

Doctor Fell was apparently a bold and resourceful
personality, quite unawed by his English colleagues.
In his remarkable letter, he made some singularly frank
and damning accusations of London physicians. He

accused them of gross cupidity and said that testimonials were available from the highest medical authorities for as little as $25.00. He charged English surgeons with operating and amputating without any justification whatsoever and said that limbs were cut off merely to satisfy the vanity or sadism of surgeons. He charged that practices were tolerated in England that would never be permitted in the United States and of all the physicians he had met in London, there were only two whom he would trust to treat himself or his family.

Despite these shocking statements, on the surface at least, Doctor Fell was on good terms with his contemporaries. Possibly he had made some mistakes in New York but had learned from them, for his conduct in London in the treatment of cancer was impeccable. Though his eventual fate is clouded in obscurity and little is known of the final years of his life, there is no evidence that he ever again fell into disgrace.

In his text on cancer,[4] published in accordance with an agreement with the Middlesex Hospital which sponsored a therapeutic test of his remedy, Doctor Fell disclosed the nature of his cancer remedy and how it should be applied, in the most ethical and conscientious manner.

The Fell remedy was derived from the root of the puccoon plant, indigenous to the shore of Lake Superior and used by the Indians for a number of different afflictions. Doctor Fell improved upon the remedy and speeded its action by the addition of chloride of zinc which he claimed enabled it to destroy large ulcerated tumors in a few weeks. The application of his preparation also required a very precise technique which was disclosed in great detail.

So careful was Doctor Fell, as he disclosed in the introductory remarks to his *Treatise*, that he kept his work in cancer a secret until he was absolutely sure his preparation had merit. Once the results were prom' ising and he was confident he could repeat his cures, he invited the leading physicians of London to wit' ness his treatments in his chambers. Over 100 doc' tors accepted his invitation and after observing his work, many commented in the most favorable terms.

Despite the letter mentioned which may have been written in a moment of pique or exasperation, Doctor Fell had no basis for complaint at the hands of his colleagues. The reception accorded him in England was one of the most unusual in the treatment of can' cer. It comprises a unique chapter in politeness and cooperation, all the more singular because Doctor Fell was on foreign soil.

When the directors of the Middlesex Hospital learned of Doctor Fell's cancer work, they courteously asked the terms upon which he would consent to an investigation. The terms were quite simple and quickly agreed upon by both sides. In return for being alloted a cancer ward at the hospital, Doctor Fell agreed to disclose in confidence to the surgical staff, the nature of his remedy, his technique of application and method of preparation. Twenty five cases were to be treated, after which Doctor Fell was obliged to publish his re' sults within six months. If he failed to publish within that period, the right fell to the board of directors.

Doctor Fell's *Treatise* consequently fulfilled his ob' ligation to the hospital. The therapeutic results of his 25 cases appeared to substantiate his claims that his treatment was far more successful than anything then available and justified abandoning surgery for relief of cancer. In an official communication, the board of directors of the Middlesex Hospital, made the following cautious endorsements of the Fell cancer treatment because

1. It was safe and conformed to surgical principles.
2. It could be employed on both operable and inoperable cancers.
3. It obviated removals of the entire breast and could be confined to enucleation of tumors only.
4. It spared patients the hazards of surgery, including hemorrhage and constitutional affections.
5. Enucleation was followed by healthy granulation and cicatrizing surface.

The board of directors withheld from their report any conclusions on the permanence of Doctor Fell's cures or the possibility of recurrences pending further observations.

Despite these highly favorable findings, the Fell remedy fell into disuse. Very little information is available on its subsequent fate, now shrouded in mystery. There is little doubt however, from the descriptions of both treatments that the Blake remedy already described, was derived from Fell's, or vice versa. Both practiced in New York at the same time and must have not only known each other but also fallen into the bad graces of the Academy of Medicine.

There is also little doubt that the Pattison therapy, whose history follows, was also identical to Fell's.

PATTISON OF LONDON

Mr. John Pattison of London was a physician with a burning independence of spirit. He, too, became embroiled with the dominating medical authorities of his day because of his outspoken opposition to the surgical treatment of cancer. The politeness accorded to Doctor Fell was denied Pattison who brought the cancer controversy to a much greater heat. Like Fell, Pattison made no secret either of his remedies or technique and freely offered to teach it to others.

Pattison published his first pamphlet on the nonsurgical treatment of cancer in 1858. In 1866 he expanded his pamphlet to a book[5] based on treating over 4,000 cancer patients in 13 years. His opponents, however, charged these cases were based on a faulty diagnostic method and he was not curing cancer but only diseases which simulated it. In rebuttal, Mr. Pattison quoted Walter Hayle Walshe, one of the greatest contemporary authorities on the disease.[6]

"Can a greater perversion of the first principles of logic exist, than that displayed by observers, who profoundly impressed with the frequent failures of all methods of cure, assume as their device the constant intractability of the disease; and when eventually obliged to admit that growths recognized as cancers, do occasionally disappear under the influence of remedies, have recourse to the plea that the disease in such instances was not really cancerous because it was cured."

In the century which had passed since Richard Guy had renounced surgery, his legitimate counterpart Pattison had inherited an evergrowing literature on the futility of surgery. To quote some of Pattison's references:

"The first and most obvious remedy is extirpating by the knife against which must be alleged the facts, that the removal of one affected part cannot remove the diathesis and that the disease is almost sure to return in the original situation or in some other.

"That the removal of the outward cancer, like the pruning of a tree, sometimes seems to raise the activity of the diathesis, and give increased energy to the morbid growth if produced afterwards. That the en tire removal of all affected particles of tissue is often unattainable. That some patients are killed by the operation itself, and that some have died from being operated on for what afterwards proved to be no cancer at all."[7]

"Of 32 cases of well-marked cancer of the breast which were operated upon by himself and 86 operated on by friends, not one was permanently cured. Several operations were fatal. He is of the opinion that the operation never corrects but almost uniformly accelerates the progress of the disease."[8]

"When malignant growths are removed with the knife, their return is but too likely,"[9]

"After amputation of a schirrous breast, under the most favorable circumstances, I believe that in ninety-nine cases out of one hundred, the disease returns."[10]

These unfavorable verdicts on surgery as a remedy for cancer were all published over a century ago. They recur repeatedly until today, despite modern improvements in technics and equipment. The dominance of surgery in the treatment of cancer despite these ominous observations has been maintained by studiously ignoring and suppressing adverse information by the powers that be.

One of the most pressing needs in cancerology is an unbiased study of the survival periods of surgical patients as compared with those who refuse surgery. Such studies are extremely rare. The most recent one is that of Hardin B. Jones,[1] but back in 1844, such a survey was compiled by Dr. Leroy-d 'Etoilles and published by the French Academy of Science. This report on cancer survival is probably the most extensive ever released. It was based on information supplied by 174 physicians on 2,781 cases, followed in some instances for over thirty years. The overall average of survival after surgery was only one year and five months.

Doctor Leroy-d 'Etiolles compiled statistics on 1,873 patients who survived an average of five years after the initial diagnosis of their cancers, classifying them according to whether they had submitted to surgery or caustics, or refused such treatment. His findings, as published in Walshe's text,[6] were:

SUMMARY OF THE LEROY-d 'ETOILLES CANCER SURVEY, 1844

Treated by Surgery or Caustics	Survival Periods			Average Survival After Initial Diagnosis	
	More than 30 Years	20 to 30 Years	6 to 20 Years	Men	Women
801	4 (12)[a]	14 (23)[a]	88 (154)[a]	5 yrs. 2 mos.	6 yrs.
Refusing Surgery or Caustics				Men	Women
1,172	18 (50%)[b]	34 (48%)[b]	228 (48%)[b]	5 yrs.	5½ yrs.

Figures in parenthesis denote:*

[a]: Number of survivors required to maintain parity in proportion to number of cases.

[b]: Greater survival value in refusing surgery or caustics, after adjustment in proportion to number of cases.

The net value of surgery or caustics, therefore, was in prolonging life two months for men and six months for women, in the first few years after the initial diagnosis. After that period, however, those who had not submitted to surgery or caustics had the greater survival potential by about 50 per cent.

Critics may say these figures prove nothing, since in all probability those who submitted to surgery or caustics were afflicted with more serious forms of cancer, while those who refused such treatment probably had less malignant cancers. The factors which enter into a decision for or against surgery or caustics are many, and probably cancel each other out. It boils down to which would arouse the greater fear—the knife, or death from cancer. Just as many patients might accept

---

* Author's analysis.

surgery because of fear of cancer as might refuse surgery because of fear of the knife, or caustics because of fear of the burning pain.

As did Richard Guy a century before him, John Pattison appraised some of the cancer remedies then in use. Arsenic had found favor because a daily ration to horses improved their endurance and gave a high gloss to their hides. After a few years, however, the continued ingestion of arsenic was found to bring on convulsions and death, not only in horses but also in humans who became addicted to it.

Some caustics then in use were nitrate of silver, quicklime, sulphate of copper (sometimes used with borax), sulfuric acid (oil of vitriol) mixed with saffron, and permanganate of pottasa. Alkaline caustics such as sulphate of zinc were also in vogue. A physician to the king of Naples had used a combination of gold, zinc and bromine which a French medical commission had investigated and rigorously condemned. Carrot poultices were also in use. The beneficial effect of these remedies in the treatment of cancer, was dubious, Mr. Pattison asserted.

His treatment demanded first that the general health of the patient be improved. Because of the constitutional nature of cancer, he prescribed a diet and also administered internal medications which he enumerated as resinous alkaloids, Polyphilin Hamamelin, Verstrun, Viride and other drugs.

Externally, Mr. Pattison applied an enucleating paste which he described openly as composed of equal parts of the powdered root of the hydrastis canadenisa, chloride of zinc, flour and water.* When properly mixed, these ingredients formed a mucilagenous mass.

---

* This formula was almost identical with Fell's.

Within from twelve to thirty-five days after the paste was applied, tumors sloughed off without bleeding, exposing a purulent mass.

According to Mr. Pattison, applying his remedy was an intricate and painstaking art, and his efforts to instruct surgeons in its use had not been altogether successful. However, he did not attribute his cures to the external application of the enucleating paste but to the constitutional treatment, with its strict diet and the elimination of salted food. For beverages, he recommended pale brandy, Hungarian Carlowitz and Tokay.

Pattison claimed his therapy was almost painless, was much safer than surgery, held a far more assuring promise of cure or alleviation and caused little shock to the system. The overwhelming dread of cancer, caused by fearful mortality from surgery was unwarranted, Mr. Pattison contended, as cancer should be treated as a constitutional disease. He offered to demonstrate his method to the directors of Middlesex Hospital in 1852 and even to work without pay. He agreed that if they would give him twenty cases, he would disclose his methods and would permit free observation and criticism of his results.

After some delay, the directors begged off, on the grounds that the hospital maintained a record of every operation in which surgeons noted unusual features of each case. In 1854, Mr. Pattison renewed his request for a test of his cancer therapy but was refused again.

Pattison consequently never enjoyed the favor accorded to his Yankee colleague, Fell. Pattison complained of being referred to sneeringly as the "cancer curer" and labeled as a quack. He also accused his colleagues of malice and using every form of chicanery to prevent cancer patients from seeking him out, even if it meant deceiving the patient.

He cited the tragic case of a woman with a growth on her breast which her physician instantly recognized as cancer but told her was benign. When she insisted upon another examination to be certain, the physician referred her to a colleague who was secretly instructed not to disclose her true condition or she would consult "that quack in London," meaning of course, Mr. Pattison. According to the latter, the referred physician obliged and removed her "benign" tumor surgically. The patient died in four weeks.

Pattison also complained his name was deliberately omitted year after year in a semiofficial directory of physicians, until an act of Parliament made the inclusion of his name mandatory. Though his status was recognized, he was never honored, for the path of the independent thinker is difficult. Mr. Pattison was outside the pale and contented himself with the gratitude of his patients. There is scant mention of his work in the official literature despite the evidence that his cancer practice was wide and extensive, possibly the greatest in London, and his results were highly beneficial.

It has just been discovered that John Pattison was originally from New York City, and like Fell, once affiliated with New York University. The strange mystery of these former Yankees practicing in London, both using an identical remedy yet hardly acknowledging each other's existence, is one of the most inexplicable in the annals of cancer. Why Fell was highly favored and Pattison persecuted is also curious and deserves investigation which at this moment, times does not permit.

CHAPTER 4

The Deficiency Approach

F. W. FORBES ROSS OF LONDON

As THE twentieth century dawned, cancer mortality rose every year. Two new discoveries, Xray and radium, were seized upon to augment surgery. The early radiologists, wholly ignorant of the powerful emanations of Xrays, were frightfully burned. Before they learned how to shield themselves while treating patients. Many technicians succumbed to cancer themselves.

About the same time, the young and brilliant physician, F. W. Forbes Ross, began practice in London. He was a born skeptic and quite independent-minded. He also wrote very wittily and gave his ideas an interesting and amusing twist in describing the foibles of mankind. Unfortunately, his career was terminated abruptly by his death at the age of forty six. In his book[11] he left a treasure of sharp and penetrating observations. Here is a sample:

"Popularly understood, 'cancer' for the lay public means something growing of a bad nature, which if not operated upon soon, that is if it can be operated upon, will cause death, and even though the sufferer submits to be 'cut up' it might return, and all the suffering will only have resulted in a short gain of time —well, one has got to go anyway."

After entering practice, Doctor Ross quickly lost faith in the orthodox cancer remedies stressed in his training and medical textbooks. He found none of any value after numerous trials. Of surgery, Xray and radium he wrote:

"A surgeon may spend his life carving his neighbor with astonishing facility and despatch, may even write a book in order to convey to the profession and his superlative success as a cutter out of cancers that can be cut out; yet, at the end of that man's life, although he has enjoyed a reputation as a good performer, he will have left nothing behind which will bring humanity, medical and lay, one iota nearer the true solution of the problem, the cause, therefore the cure of cancer. . . .

"When Roentgen discovered the Xray whilst experimenting with a Crookes tube . . . a few enterprising medical souls decided that Xray might be useful in the treatment of cancer. It was immediately adopted and became the law of the medical Medes and Persians for inoperable cases of cancer, simply because the so-called 'cancer experts'—who as operative curers had failed and were at their wits end to find some feasible excuse and method with which to cover their paralyzed resources—had decided to adopt Xrays. The first trial of Xrays as a treatment of cancer was the blindest of blind leaps in the dark by even the most orthodox." [11]

The same blind embrace of radium followed its discovery by the Curies. There was no doubt of the power of its emanations, and power is always held in awe; but just what those emanations comprised or how they worked was not clear. According to Doctor Ross:

"Why Xray and radium are supposed to act beneficially was supposed to be on account of their ultra violet (alpha, beta, gamma) rays. What particular process or action these rays exerted, no one knew. Why Xray or radium should influence some growths and cause growths in others, no one knew." [11]

When Doctor Ross began his lamentably short ca-reer, he followed the consensus of cancer experts in those days that the disease was infectious and was caused by microorganisms or psorosperms.* They rec-ommended salicylate of soda, quinine, salicylic acid, carbolic acid, mercury, iodine, arsenic and other drugs to combat the cancer germ. Ross found these remedies ineffectual; if there was a cancer germ, it survived the attacks of all the textbook germicides he prescribed.

Not content to continue prescribing these dubious official remedies, even though protected from criticism by adhering to orthodoxy, Doctor Ross began his own researches. Disregarding everything he had been taught, he started from the very beginning with a thorough study of the physiology, anatomy and chemistry of the cancer cell.

Through a series of interesting and scientific de-ductions, Doctor Ross arrived at the theory that can-cer is caused by a deficiency of some vital substance which enable the healthy cell to maintain its proper form and function. In cancer, this regulating power to duplicate the cells properly is lost because of the lack of that vital biochemical element. Malformed and widely proliferating cells, completely out of control, then replace the normal cells.

After studying the chemical functioning of the en-docrine glands, the blood and the over-all nutritional requirements of the human system, Doctor Ross iden-tified potassium salts as the missing element which

---

* The virus theory dating back over 60 years has had a checkered history in cancer. Once it was the rage but in the early decades of the twentieth century it was discredited and practically banned. It has been revived again in recent years and is now so respectable that 1956 Dr. Wendell M. Stanley of the University of California received a Nobel prize for his studies on the cancer virus.

maintains normal cell life. He insisted that these salts were increasingly being processed out of foods; that there was deficiency in foods because the soil was being depleted of essential minerals; and that in cooking vegetables and meats, even more of these precious salts were lost. As a result, food ingested was seriously deficient in needed elements.

In the treatment of cancer, Doctor Ross prescribed potassium citrate and phosphate to correct the mineral deficiency, with a weekly dose of five grains of potassium iodide. His cancer patients were either the hopeless and inoperable or those who had refused surgery or irradiation. In a number of these cases adjudged as hopeless, he was remarkably successful. He prescribed potassium routinely to all his other patients and claimed that over a period fifteen years no patient under his care had contracted cancer.

The Ross therapy was aimed at correcting the general well-being of the cancer patient and at bringing back the natural color of the hair and skin by improving the dietary intake. With the return of general bodily health, the tumor usually began to recede. Doctor Ross also found that the average cancer patient had certain uniform predilections for food. As a rule, they habitually ate rich and spicy foods, were primarily meat eaters, disliked vegetables and rarely drank the water in which vegetables were cooked. They also preferred distilled liquors to wine and beer, which are malt products and generally retain their potassium. In studying the diet of healthy, primitive races, Doctor Ross learned that they avoided such eating practices and that their diets included only raw and fresh foods, with all nutrients retained.

Believing that no disease could be corrected until the body's natural functions were restored, the Ross therapy consequently consisted in restoring the natural protective substances in foods and since a cancer cure must provide all the nutritive elements present in good, fresh foods, his therapy also included a dietary education for cancer patients.

There have been many nutritional discoveries since Doctor Ross's, but none of his ideas and principles has become obsolete. The degeneration of processed foods and the addition of carcinogenic chemical preservatives and adulterants is greater today that it was fifty years ago. Cancer is also more prevalent, consistently confirming the correctness of the Ross approach.

It is significant that practically every cancer therapist who abandoned surgery and irradiation recognized the curative value of proper diet. It is also true that the socalled "official school" regarded such thinking with deeper and deeper aversion. To stress the nutritional approach to cancer eventually became the surest way to become branded as a quack.

Doctor Ross suffered some of that anathema, although he was a mild heretic, as heretics in diet go. He did not exclude meat, tea, coffee and malt liquors from the diet, and he believed that surgery had some place in cancer and that radium could be beneficial if the potassium level was maintained by doubling consumption, since Xrays deplete the patient's potassium reserves.

To demonstrate how dangerous it was to differ from orthodox opinions, Ross cited the case of a physician who, during the era when tuberculosis was regarded as fatal and incurable, dared to suggest that it was curable.

"What!" thundered a leading power in the medical profession in an open medical meeting. "Did I hear

you correctly? Have you the temerity to say that consumption can be cured?"

The heretic was steadfast in his heresy, only to be
broken and ruined by an "important medical body,"
according to Forbes Ross.

Cancer may now be going through the same history
as many diseases formerly considered incurable, such
as typhoid fever, tuberculosis, scurvy, smallpox and
pneumonia. Today few diseases are considered incurable; cancer is one of these rare exceptions. The cures
were for the most part discovered by men who dared
to be in advance of their times. In practically every
instance, new discoveries were at first bitterly assailed,
only to win grudging approval later.

The same is true in cancer. For many years the only
therapy recognized by the entrenched powers were
surgery and irradiation. The recent renascence of the
virus theory and the presently curative hopes in a
chemotherapeutic approach herald the acceptance of
ideas that were fairly stated many years ago by pioneers like F. W. Forbes Ross and others whose work
will be described.

ROBERT BELL, EX-SURGEON

Robert Bell was another English heretical physician
of great integrity. He, too, became embroiled with the
medical hierarchy when he abandoned surgery for cancer and militantly campaigned against the knife. Originally from Glasgow, Doctor Bell moved to London,
where he practiced medicine for over half a century.
His career from 1894, when he abandoned surgery for
cancer, until his death in 1928 was an adventurous
struggle replete with many battles in his crusade for
a nonsurgical approach to cancer.

Doctor Bell practiced surgery with great skill until 1894, when he realized his results in the surgery of cancer had been very poor and he gave it up. An idea of his attainments may be gained from a resume of his contributions to medical science apart from can' cer therapy. In 1872, Bell was elected a Fellow in the Royal Faculty of Physicians and Surgeons; in the 1870's he devised an improved method of treating diphtheria and an improvement in treating smallpox which elim' inated the secondary fever. In the 1880's he identified constipation as a cause of disease and named the re' sulting absorption of toxic material into the blood "au' totoxemia." He also originated the microphotograph; he perfected the technique by working late at night when all traffic was stilled as the slightest vibration would spoil his plates. In his autobiography,[12] he re' produced a few of his exquisite woodcuts of photo' micography.

After abandoning surgery, Doctor Bell advocated the correction of constipation and the adoption of a vegetarian diet which retained the original nutrients in the foods. In 1896 he read a paper before the British Gynecological Society advancing dietary approaches to cancer and deploring the disastrous effects of surgery. His stormy and militant career can be traced from that address. Such views inevitably led to bitter contro' versies with his colleagues and eventually involved the doughty Bell in several law suits and investigations.

He read the same paper before the International Gynecology Society that year, but the surgeons again refused to take heed. In 1899 he read it again before the same society at an Amsterdam meeting. A famous surgeon there listened, but said not a word although Doctor Bell charged that two patients upon whom that surgeon had operated upon for cancer had died shortly before in frightful agony. Moreover, the same surgeon continued to operate on tumors despite continued lamentable results.

In 1903, Doctor Bell published the first edition of his masterpiece *The Treatment of Cancer without Operation*.[13] The New York *Medical Record* gave it an impartial review, but in England it met a scathing and denunciatory reception.

This was understandable for Doctor Bell had continually assailed the shocking amount of error in diagnosing cancer and the over readiness of surgeons to wield the knife. He charged that inflamed breasts, too often only symptomatic of mastitis, were ruthlessly removed when proper medication would have resulted in healing within three to four weeks.

One case he cited was that of a woman whose milk overflowed. The condition was diagnosed as cancer. Doctor Bell contended that a cancerous breast could not give milk. After the woman was operated upon, a cancer did develop and she died three months after the birth of her child.

Doctor Bell charged that surgeons were prone to remove every lump in the breast as cancerous, whereas at least half of all breast tumors were not malignant and would yield to other types of therapy. Surgery on nonmalignant tumors actually incited the development of a malignancy, he contended, pointing to the alarming increase in cancer from 63.0 per 100,000 population in 1900 to 79.4 in 1914 which attended the wider use of surgery.

King Edward recognized Doctor Bell's unusual energy and talents despite the controversies that raged about him, and offered him a title. Bell was forced to decline, for the title would have necessitated outlays which he was unable to make because his practice was not sufficiently lucrative.

In 1912, Doctor Bell was violently attacked in the *British Medical Journal* by Dr. E. V. Bashford, general superintendent of the Imperial Cancer Fund, who called him a quack. In a suit for libel which he quickly instituted, Doctor Bell was awarded £2,000 ($10,000).

Doctor Bell's enemies also tried to make capital of a woman who had died of cancer under his care. The circumstances were typical of his willingness to help the unfortunate. The patient had been unable to pay, and he had undertaken her treatment after her own physician had failed to help her and had refused further cooperation on the case. Doctor Bell's treatment consisted only of general instructions on diet and hygiene.

The woman succumbed some nine months later, whereupon the Council of Physicians received a complaint from her husband. The Council demanded an explanation from Doctor Bell while at the same time refusing to name the source of the complaint. Only after a writ was obtained to force this disclosure did they comply.

The inquiry which followed completely exonerated Doctor Bell. The first physician in the case was the one who was really culpable. He had watched the woman go from bad to worse; and even after she had received Doctor Bell's advice, which was of a general nature and could not possibly have done her any harm, he had rendered no cooperation whatsoever. To exemplify the irony of the matter. Doctor Bell claimed that had he left the woman to her fate for fear of criticism, there would have been no action against him.

But it was Doctor Bell's fate to suffer such prosecution despite his superlative competence and integrity. He was refused permission to submit papers to the

Royal Society of Medicine and was compelled to publish them independently.

One baffling question which he clarified was whether
tumors could result from blows or continued irritation. In recent years the injury or irritation theory
has been discredited on the grounds that most people
suffer injuries at some time, yet a vast majority of
them do not contract cancer.

Doctor Bell believed that injuries are a factor in
the development of cancer. In healthy tissue, he reasoned blood resulting from internal bleeding is quickly
absorbed without leaving clots. Clotting is necessary
only to seal an external wound. In an acute or sub-
acute inflammatory condition, however, the tissue cannot absorb blood. A hard, internal clot which may
therefore result acts somewhat like a foreign body and
become the nucleus of a tumor.

The factor of injury and irritation as a cause of
cancer has been bruited about for many decades, but
Doctor Bell's is the most lucid and ingenious explanation yet offered. His theory makes it clear that cancer can result both from a general constitutional disability with attendant inflamed tissues becoming ag-
gravated by local irritations or injuries. Internal
bleeding also does not necessarily result from injuries
or irritations alone but may be caused by fragile blood
vessels and capillaries, also an unhealthy constitutional
condition.

The Bell explanation accounts as well for the recurrence of cancers at the site of incisions because of
the adherence of blood clots which cause tumor growths.

Doctor Bell also pointed to the high proportion of
myxedema (low functioning thyroid conditions) in
cancer. He advocated curing cancer by restoring the
thyroid gland to normal functioning. In recent years

this observation has been confirmed by Dr. G. W. Crile, Jr., of the Cleveland Clinic, who states that hypothyroidism should not be allowed to exist in cancer patients and that recurrences of cancer have been avoided by the administration of thyroid extract.[14]

Doctor Bell's career affirms the evidence that the fate of the cancer heretic, regardless of his qualifications and past achievements, whether he be the recipient of high medical honors or without medical qualifications of any kind, is equally unpleasant. The inevitable results have been accusations of quackery, followed by ostracism.

LUCIUS DUNCAN BULKLEY OF NEW YORK

In the United States, Dr. Robert Bell had a worthy contemporary in his warm friend, Dr. Lucius Duncan Bulkley of New York City. The experiences and personalities of the two men were remarkably similar. Both made distinguished contributions to medicine during long and honorable careers. Both were incapable of subterfuge. Both strongly opposed the surgical treatment of cancer. Both advocated the constitutional, dietetic approach in cancer treatment.

Doctor Bulkley was the son of a renowned physician. After an excellent training both in the United States and Europe, he specialized in dermatology, as his father had before him. He wrote a number of extensive works and articles on skin diseases and soon attained the reputation of an authority in that field.

Cancerology and dermatology are quite closely associated, and in 1885 Doctor Bulkley was instrumental in organizing the New York Skin and Cancer Hospital, which he served as a director for many years. He was allotted a ward with twelve beds, and he also directed an out patient clinic devoted exclusively to cancer patients.

Doctor Bulkley, too, became deeply convinced that dietary factors in cancer patients must be carefully regulated, and he prescribed a strict vegetarian diet. He also believed that constipation was a causative factor, and always instituted measures to correct it.

The tenor of his opposition to surgery can be judged from the following quotations:

"Surgeons claim that an early operation secures a successful result. This is by no means true, for we have seen plenty instances of excellent operations by highly competent operators immediately on the first discovery of the lesion, in which there were serious after results and even death. . . .

"It is now generally agreed that a biopsy in cancer is always a very questionable procedure as it tends to spread the disease and to render the prognosis unfavorable, and it would be especially perilous in such cases about to undergo medical treatment, and would not be at all justified simply to satisfy so-called scientific curiosity or doubt. My long experience has shown me that the more biopsies there are, the more necropsies there are."[15]

Doctor Bulkley was extremely well read, and his books and papers are liberally interspersed with quotations from leading authorities of different eras. He cited the greatest teachers as far back as John Abernethy, the renowned English surgeon, who earnestly wrote in 1816 that cancer was a constitutional disease not confined to the local growth and should be so regarded.

In 1844, Walshe had already written: "it would in theory appear that the removal of a tumor cannot of itself cure the disease, as the local formation is but a symptom of a general vice of the economy."[6]

To prove the futility of surgery, Doctor Bulkley pointed to the ever-increasing cancer mortality despite the dominance of surgery. In 1900, cancer deaths were 63 per 100,000 population; in 1915, 81.1; in 1927, 103.

He also cited the consequences of an active propaganda campaign for cancer surgery, directed to the public in the early nineteen twenties. A year after that campaign, cancer deaths had doubled over the average for the previous five years. In contrast, Doctor Bulkley cited the fact that there was a steady decline in tuberculosis because of the educational campaign for improved diet and sanitation as a preventive. The contagious nature of tuberculosis had acted powerfully to arouse the public but unfortunately, he observed, this spur could not be used in cancer because it was not contagious.

Doctor Bulkley also criticised the futility of animal experimentation in cancer research.* He urged that clinical and laboratory studies of human cancer were of far greater value. Prolonged studies of the metabolism of cancer patients invariably showed marked departures from the normal, he contended, thus confirming Bell's observation that the thyroid was often deeply involved in cancer. Departure from normal metabo-

---

* Time has borne out Doctor Bulkley's opinion, judging from the following statement of the French authority, Charles Oberling:

"The animal bearing a transplanted neoplasm . . . is but a cultural medium for cells that are not his own, and toward which he consequently re-acts in a totally different way.

"As a result, interest in the questions that transplantable tumors were once expected to solve has inevitably fallen off, for more must never be demanded of a method than it can give. Altogether they have turned out to be a grand illusion for so little do they resemble the spontaneous new growth that they are utterly incapable of furnishing information applicable to man, or of providing the least insight into the cause of the malignant change, since they were already established from the first." [16]

lism was detected by Doctor Bulkley from evidence in the blood, skin, feces and urine and from analyses of the salivary and possibly the endocrine secretions.

Some surgeons privately acknowledged the justice of Doctor Bulkley's criticism of surgery. He quoted an outstanding tumor surgeon of New Jersey as having confessed: "I have done with operations on cancer and hope that no one will ever again ask me to op- erate on that disease. I do not know that I have ever done enough good to warrant the operation."

From his own practice, Doctor Bulkley published the results of his treatment of 250 cases of breast can- cer without surgery.[17] He was able to demonstrate sufficient alleviation and prolongation of life, without undue suffering, to justify his procedure. Many of his patients had confided to him that they had suffered more anguish from the continual worry caused by the warnings of friends or physicians that they must un- dergo surgery than they had from the disease or its treatment.

This adamant opposition to surgery eventually led to the abolishment of Doctor Bulkley's special ward and clinic at the New York Skin and Cancer Hos- pital, when the board of directors decreed that hence- forth surgery would be the treatment of choice. When Cancer and its Non-Surgical Treatment was reviewed later that year (1921) in the Journal of the American Medical Association, a letter from the board of gov- ernors of the hospital was also published, regretting "that the name of the hospital had been associated with this and similar publications which so completely misrepresent its policies."

Another ironic circumstance in Doctor Bulkley's life was the sad fate of his own son-in-law, Dr. H. H. Janeway, one of the founders of Memorial Hos-

pital and a pioneer in radium treatment. Doctor Janeway died of cancer of the face at an early age, despite fourteen operations and many years of suffering
and pain.

Doctor Bulkley died in 1928. He left a monument
to his distinguished career in a treasure of sage, honest
and penetrating observations. His nutritional approach
to the cure of cancer and his opposition to surgery,
biopsies and pure animal experimentation appear to
be as valid as ever and deserve renewed interest in
the light of current trends.

THE OZIAS TREATMENT

About the turn of the century, Charles Othello
Ozias, M.D., of Nevada, Missouri, became engaged
in the treatment of cancer. According to the auto-
biographical reference in his book, he was born and
raised on a farm. He knew the joys and hardships
of farm life, and attributed the robust health and vigor
of farm people to their strenuous toil and the nourish-
ing quality of their home-grown foods. He blamed
modern illnesses on the softness of city life and on
its devitalized, denatured foods. Doctor Ozias prescribed natural, health-giving foods in his cancer treatment, together with a medicament whose nature he
would not disclose. This put him in the category of
using a secret remedy, which may have been the preparation mentioned in this passage from his book:

"About a third of a century ago, an eminent specialist practicing in the East confided to me that the
aqueous solution of Secalae Cornutum injected hypo-
dermically into the thyroid gland would cure goiter.
Successfully following that method of procedure in
many cases for several years, I was impressed that

something should be done on this plan for our women to correct the abnormal condition of the ovary and diseases affecting the same."[18]

This preparation may have hormonal properties and consequently could be of benefit in cancer. At any rate, Doctor Ozias became so celebrated for his cancer cures that he built his own hospital in Kansas City, Missouri. In 1922 he wrote to the American Medical Association and to local medical societies in several states, offering to treat one hundred cases free of charge in his hospital and to disclose his formula for distribution to the medical profession if the results of his treatment were published in one of the official AMA journals. His offer was not accepted, but Doctor Ozias soon found himself repeatedly brought into court, which required much time and money for his defense. Time after time he was indicted, but the case was withdrawn before a decision was rendered. This finally bankrupted the doctor and he was forced to give up his hospital. He retired to his old house in Nevada, Missouri, where he carried on a greatly restricted practice until he died.

In 1942, Doctor Ozias told his story to a physician visiting him to observe his cancer therapy. On his first visit to Doctor Ozias, then seventy-nine years old, the visiting physician was permitted to examine three cancer patients. He found extensive involvement with severe symptoms of toxicity. Three weeks later he was allowed to examine the patients again, and he stated in a letter: "All three had made almost complete recovery so far as symptoms of palpable growth masses were concerned. It was the most amazing thing I have ever seen in rapid improvement in cancer cases."

The physician, whose name cannot be revealed, attempted to secure the Ozias formula but was refused.

The aged doctor was so bitter because of the treatment meted out to him that he vowed never to give away his secret. When he died several years later, the formula may have died with him.

In the early 1930's, however, Norman Baker of Muscatine, Iowa, the notorious figure who broadcast on many controversial issues over his own radio station, learned of the Ozias cancer therapy. He sent several patients to Dr. Ozias and was so impressed with the results that he got the notion to establish his own clinic and to engage physicians to dispense the Ozias treatment as his own. Baker advertised his cancer cures in his newspaper and over his radio station. Patients began to flock to Muscatine but it was not long until the AMA began its attack.

A little later, Harry M. Hoxsey and Dr. Bruce Miller were also engaged by Baker. This association lasted only five months. Hoxsey avers that Baker was greedy and raised his fees, but refused to spend money to expand the clinic's facilities as the patients flocked there or to treat those unable to pay the high fees.

Baker eventually lost his broadcasting license but established another radio station just over the Mexican border to give him access to United States listeners. In 1940 he established a cancer clinic in Little Rock, Arkansas, but after he was convicted of unethical practices, the clinic was closed. In 1944 Baker was released from prison and retired to live on a yacht. He was possibly one of the most unsavory figures in the history of cancer quackery, although the treatment he used did have merit because it was originated by Doctor Ozias.

As this work goes to press, it is reported that Norman Baker died.

CHAPTER 5

Toxins, Serums, Hormones

THE COLEY TOXINS

In 1891, W. B. Coley, M.D., of New York City, began employing fever incitants in the treatment of cancer. Until he died in 1936, he devoted himself entirely to that approach with fair success. Today a few disciples still carry on his work by seeking toxins of greater and greater reliability for inducing fevers in cancer patients.

Doctor Coley's interest in cancer originated when a patient with bone sarcoma expired under his care after repeated operations. He determined then and there to concentrate upon finding a cure for the disease, and studied all reported cases of bone sarcoma dating from 1876. Then, one day in 1891, he was confronted with another case.

Three times he operated without success. The patient then contracted erysipelas, a highly dangerous and infectious inflammatory skin disease accompanied by high fever. After recovering from one attack, he suffered another with the attending fever. After the second attack, the patient not only recovered from the erysipelas, but his bone sarcoma also disappeared.

That was an instance of nature herself curing, of a disease curing a disease. Fascinated by the spontaneous cure he had observed, Doctor Coley spent the rest of his career trying to duplicate nature's method of healing by fever. He was not the first, however, to stumble across the phenomenon, although he was the most persistent in trying to duplicate it.

In 1866, William Busch of Bonn, a Prussian physician, had also observed a remission of cancer following an attack of erysipelas. In 1910, Tuffier, a French physician, had cured an actress of cancer by inducing an artificial fever, but he failed to duplicate his success with other patients because they became tolerant to fever incitants and he could not sustain the necessary high internal temperature.

Doctor Coley encountered the same difficulties for many years, but he persisted and experimented constantly with different dosages in the search for more effective toxins. He found that increasing the dosage to almost prohibitive levels, at times, brought on fevers of sufficient intensity and duration to heal cancer.

The administration of the Coley toxins however, required great patient and skill. Christian and Palmer reported attaining success with the toxins under circumstances that Doctor Coley himself confessed he would not have persevered. It was a case of cancer which had developed in the stump of an amputated leg. The two physicians administered the toxins for several months without discernible results when suddenly the fever took hold and eventually eradicated the cancer.[19]

While the Coley toxins have occasionally been successful, the number and proportion of cures has not been spectacular. In seeking the still undiscovered ideal toxin, fourteen different preparations have been tried with varying success. The criticism of the Coley toxins is based on the difficulty of deciding when they should be administered in preference to other treatments and because of the many failures reported when it was used.

Research with the Coley toxins is continued today by the New York Cancer Institute. According to the Institute's published conclusions[20] the increasing incidence of cancer, even after allowing for exaggerations because of improper diagnosis, coincides with the introduction of asepsis and public health measures for the prevention of contagious disease. With lessened exposure to infection has come lessened ability to cope with disease. This opinion is also shared by G. Jacobson, a German authority. He attributed the decline in disease resistance to lessened exposure to infection and the resulting inactivity of the reticulo-endothelial system, which creates immunity to disease.

The immunity created by infection has also been observed in leukemia by M. J. Shear. He reported 75 per cent of leukemia following attacks of acute diseases.[21] However, it appears that this promising clue has not been followed very vigorously.

Although Doctor Coley's work did not meet the bitter opposition of many other independent approaches, neither did it receive much encouragement. In 1934 the *Journal of the American Medical Association* published some faint praise of the Coley toxins as one of the "very few" cancer nostrums with some merit. There is a prevailing but false idea in the medical profession that the Coley toxins are specific only for bone tumors, whereas actually such tumors are more resistant to them. This false notion arose because Doctor Coley was once active in the bone tumor service at Memorial Hospital.

Doctor Coley's work is also interesting from another stand-point—the virus theory of cancer. As far back as 1893, he stated that both sarcoma and carcinoma could be attributed to some microbic or virus origin and in 1929 reaffirmed that this belief was strongly supported by clinical evidence. In view of the recent interest in the virus theory, after many years of neg- lect and indifference, this statement is extremely in- teresting:

"Why is it that in so many of the great cancer research institutions of the world this question of the parasitic origin of cancer receives practically no atten- tion today? It is because no young man entering the field of cancer research feels that he can afford to run the risk of an unsympathetic and often antagonistic attitude on the part of professors of pathology who repeatedly tell him that the whole matter has been definitely settled and that cancer cannot possibly be of germ origin . . . I urge once more that we look upon the theory of a microbic cause of cancer not as a closed chapter, but one that deserves sympathetic study. Every encouragement should be given to work- ers in this field."[22]

THE COFFEY-HUMBER EXTRACT

The controversy attending the development and pub- licizing of the Coffey-Humber extract for the treatment of cancer which culminated in its rejection deserves the most careful study. As I attempted to testify at the California hearings, this seething dispute over the merits of a cancer nostrum of the early 1930's is an ideal example of how controversies originate follow- ing publicity and how frantically patients respond to the slightest hopes of a new remedy.

The Coffey-Humber extract is no longer sponsored, but it was once endorsed by very influential interests and had the advantages of liberal financial backing, ex- tensive clinical testing, widespread publicity and highly capable scientific development. Yet, withal, it was strongly opposed by powerful interests. Eventually it was ignored and discarded with hardly the semblance of fair scientific and clinical test, if such a test can be said to exist in appraising cancer remedies.

Dr. Walter B. Coffey, who died in 1944, was chief surgeon and director of the Southern Pacific Railroad Hospital in San Francisco from 1926 to 1938. Almost his entire professional career was spent in the service of the railroad either in a full-time or part-time capacity. He was highly respected for his surgical skill, and in the 1920's originated an operation to relieve the intense pain of angina pectoris; he was invited to demonstrate his technique before several leading universities in Europe.

It was during this period that Doctor Coffey became interested in cancer therapy. According to a newspaper story, he experimented with an adrenal extract in treating high blood pressure in a patient who was also cancerous. The extract not only dramatically relieved the high blood pressure, but the cancer as well. Dr. Coffey then claimed that, together with Dr. John D. Humber, he had experimented with various extracts from the adrenal cortex of cattle until he derived one from sheep which seemed most effective.

I was fortunate in being able to meet a San Francisco physician who had known Doctor Coffey quite well and who had some "inside information" which differs somewhat from newspaper stories. This physician stated that the adrenal preparation was not Dr. Coffey's discovery at all but had originally been prepared by the late Doctor Eaton, a celebrated San Francisco urologist. Eaton had himself been encouraged by Gye the English cancerologist, to investigate the hormones of the adrenal cortex.

When Doctor Coffey learned of Eaton's work, according to my informant, he appropriated it as his own. As a consequence there was bad feeling on Doctor Eaton's part. As the director of a large hospital, Doctor Coffey was in an ideal position to test the extract, and when sufficient clinical evidence was available he made a demonstration before the San Francisco Pathological Society in January, 1930, for which he received wide publicity. Reporters described the astonishment of some patients at their improvement. Some with stomach cancer said they were again able to retain food after receiving injections of the Coffey-Humber extract. There were numerous expressions about decreased pain and a general improvement in health.

Many prominent physicians commented in highly favorable terms. A noted surgeon from Seattle called the extract "the greatest discovery in the field of medicine." Another said enthusiastically that there was "nothing like it; even if it was not a specific cure it was a remarkable means to lessen unbearable pain." Dr. George H. Kress, dean of the Los Angeles branch of the University of California, extolled Doctor Coffey's "brilliance and fast, accurate thinking." He added: "We are not surprised that so important a beginning of anti-cancer work should come from him." There was a rising ovation for Doctor Coffey from over 1,200 California physicians at their convention in 1930.

As a result of the publicity, Doctor Coffey was besieged by cancer patients. He announced in the press the conditions of acceptance for treatment, which required a letter from the referring physicians certifying that cancer had been diagnosed by approved laboratory procedures and that the patient could not be helped further by surgery or irradiation. Only inoperable cancers would be treated; operable cases and

those suitable for irradiation treatment were unacceptable. Patients from distant points and those in a dying
condition were also discouraged from seeking treatment. In the interests of science, those accepted for
treatment were asked to agree to an autopsy if they
succumbed.

This publicity was repugnant to Morris Fishbein,
then editor of the AMA *Journal,* who editorialized:

"Pathologists and surgeons who have investigated
the method express nothing but profound disappoint-
ment with both the clinical and pathological results.
These experts indicate that post-mortem examinations
which have been made in at least 30 cases do not reveal any definite specific destruction of cancer tissue
or evidence that the spread of cancer in the bodies of
the afflicted patients has been retarded."

At their annual meeting, members of the California
State Medical Society criticized Morris Fishbein for
these "unethical and unscientific" remarks. Doctor
Coffey replied through the press:

"It appears highly unjust and unethical if Doctor
Fishbein has employed pathologists working in secret.
Such investigations could have been carried on openly
at any of our clinics with our utmost cooperation.
Secret investigations such as he implies remind one of
the secret tribunals of medieval days when the accused
was tried and sentenced without opportunity to defend himself at open trial."

Publicity became nation wide. Not all of it was
favorable. One physician stated that he had observed
the application of the extract for three weeks without
seeing any encouraging results. Others deplored the
raising of false hopes in cancer sufferers with an un-
proved, dubious remedy; they discouraged prospective
patients from mortgaging their homes to go to Cal-

ifornia for treatment with the extract. According to another critic, research organizations had experimented for years with adrenal hormones without finding anything hopeful.

Nevertheless, patients by the thousands flocked to the Coffey-Humber Cancer Clinic. A branch was opened in Los Angeles, and in 1931 permission was sought from the New York State Welfare Board to open a clinic in New York City. The wealthy widow of a railroad magnate offered to donate her magnificent million-dollar mansion on Long Island for the use of a Coffey-Humber clinic.

Opposition rose in full force against granting this permission. Hearings were held in New York City, at which the Coffey-Humber interests were represented by Herbert Satterlee, attorney for J. P. Morgan and Company, bankers for the Southern Pacific Railroad. Mr. Satterlee decried the "Chinese wall of opposition" erected against the Coffey-Humber extract, but in spite of his plea the Welfare Board refused to sanction opening of the clinic.

Later that year, under the auspices of the Kellogg Foundation, Dr. Rowland H. Harris reported in the *Journal* of the AMA that he had investigated the extract and found it worthless if not harmful. In some instances, he wrote, injections accelerated the growth of tumors. Dr. R. W. Starr, director of the Los Angeles Coffey-Humber Cancer Clinic, accused Doctor Harris of supplying a false report and of not keeping his records in accordance with their agreement, as it was impossible to determine from his findings how many patients had died of diseases other than cancer. Doctor Starr also appended clinical studies of a number of cases Doctor Harris had studied but not reported, although they had shown marked improvement.

In March, 1936, Doctor Coffey and Humber published their results with 7,513 presumably hopeless cancer patients.[23] Of these, 3,872 died before they could receive 30 injections, the minimum considered necessary for a fair test. Out of 1,040 cases treated adequately, about 10 per cent lived four or more years. Doctor Coffey claimed that this was a significant and commendable result in the light of the statement of the eminent pathologist Ewing that not 5 per cent recovered from cancer after surgery or irradiation.

This claim had also been made by Doctor Coffey at the annual meeting of the American College of Surgeons in 1933, but it was received with indifference if not antipathy. Balfour, the noted surgeon of the Mayo Clinic, was quoted in *Time* as saying: "Cancer is curable if removed while it is a local disease. Cures by advertised serums, extracts, etc., are myths."

Interest in and support for the Coffey-Humber extract gradually declined until complete silence ensued. Doctor Coffey died in 1944. Doctor Humber who is still in practice, stated over the telephone that he no longer uses the extract.

Regardless of its merits, the remedy was never scientifically investigated by opponents. The clinical trials however were very competently and accurately conducted and observed by qualified physicians. The criticism of the Kellogg Foundation report as unfair, since it was based only on the examination of records which were inaccurately compiled, seems well founded.

Widely conflicting opinions are the rule in cancer controversies. Doctor Garland, the radiologist, testified at the California hearings that he was well acquainted with the Coffey-Humber extract; that, according to the charts of nurses, it did not relieve pain; and that he saw patients "die like flies."

But only terminal cases were treated in the first place. Doctor Coffey wrote that the patients with the poorest response to his extract were those who had been treated extensively by irradiation, which seemed to deplete their recuperative powers.

So the matter rests. In spite of the vast amounts of time and money spent testing the Coffey-Humber extract, nothing conclusive has ever been reported. Even a negative finding based on sound scientific evidence would be valuable as a safeguard against similar experiments in the future. Whether or not the Coffey-Humber extract had alleviative powers, or at least was helpful in relieving pain and eliminating the need for narcotics, is still a mystery.

THE GLOVER ANTI-CANCER SERUM

Another great mystery in the history of cancer is the fate of Glover's cancer serum once widely publicized as having great promise. It was developed by Dr. Thomas J. Glover and several associates whose scientific studies were meticulously and competently carried out. Reports were duly published in various medical journals about thirty years ago, but are now almost forgotten. The recent renascence of the virus theory of cancer makes these forgotten Glover researches of great interest.

Soon after entering medical practice in 1911 in Toronto, Canada, where he continues to practice today, Dr. Thomas J. Glover was attracted to the study of cancer viruses. Financed by a wealthy industrialist, he developed a serum derived from the blood of horses. It was found promising and was donated to hospitals for clinical testing, in accordance with the usual procedure.

After encouraging reports from hospital clinics,

Doctor Glover became widely known and was besieged by cancer patients from all over North America. His fame enabled him to move from a modest home to a luxurious residence, according to a newspaper story. The events following his ascent to recognition and affluence are typical in the history of cancer remedies developed by independent workers, for in 1921 the Toronto Academy of Medicine appointed a special committee to conduct the inevitable investigation. The committee's report of January 13, 1921, reads in part:

"From the data so far obtained the committee has found no evidence to warrant the hope that a specific cure for cancer has been discovered by Doctor Glover, or that a cure has been produced by the serum in any case definitely established as cancer. The data which your committee has been able to obtain have not convinced it that results of treatment obtained by the use of Glover's serum are better than those obtained by similar methods introduced by others and which have ultimately failed the hopes obtained for them."

The committee also reported that Doctor Glover refused to allow its members to visit his laboratory or to examine his experimental material. The investigators also believed that some apparent cures of Doctor Glover were the result of psychic suggestion and would have no lasting effects.

Nevertheless, a number of physicians both in Canada and the United States became interested in the Glover serum. In 1923 a comprehensive report was prepared for the Philadelphia *North American,* but the article was withheld from publication for fifteen months "in the interests of science," as the New York *Times* put it. On June 4, 1924, the article was finally published. It kicked up quite a storm. According to the *Times,* the report covered work conducted for four

years. After the serum had proved effective upon animals inoculated with carcinoma, it was injected in
cancer patients at several leading Philadelphia hospitals. In two years the serum was administered to more
than two hundred cases of confirmed cancer representing every stage of the disease from incipient and localized to terminal and metastatic. Nearly one hundred of these cases were confined at the National Stomach Hospital, and a majority were reported to have
responded favorably.

The decided bias against the virus theory of cancer,
as mentioned by Doctor Coley, became evident in the
strong opposition against acceptance of the report. The
day following its publication, the great Ewing was
quoted in the New York Times:

"There is no microorganismal cause of cancer and
as soon as the public learns this fact, the less likely will
they be deceived by claims such as those Doctor Glover
makes. As cancer is not a germborn disease, a serum
treatment would be worthless. The effective treatment
of cancer is accomplished by surgery, the Xray and
radium in combination.

"The cure of cancer otherwise than by surgery depends upon the discovery of its cause and that remains
as yet a mystery, through which only a few gleams of
doubtful light have been cast."

The opposition was evidently determined to protect
the public from the consequences of being misled into
believing the virus theory of cancer. On June 11, the
day following, the New York Times published an editorial stating that Doctor Glover had announced from
San Francisco, where he was attending a medical congress, that claims made in his behalf for the curative
powers of his serum were "premature" and that he
himself would make no further statements until he had

something to report to his colleagues. The editorial then continued:

"While it is evident the medical profession is not ready to admit Doctor Glover's claims, his repudiation should mitigate the severity of any criticisms because he promptly repudiated claims made in his behalf . . .

"There is nothing in the Glover or any other cancer cure to warrant delaying surgery for a single day."

Evidently Doctor Glover's repudiation either was not geniune or was falsely reported, for less than a month later he renewed his claims before the Philadelphia Clinical Society, in his paper, "The Etiology of Cancer—Treatment of Cancer with Antibacterial and Antitoxic Serum." He presented a complete description of the microorganisms he believed to be the cause of cancer, as well as proof of results obtained with his antiserum in a number of pathologically confirmed cases.

Again the opposition raged against Glover who later wrote of his opponents: "The antagonism displayed by several medical men, in denouncing the facts presented without even a pretext at investigation, is to be regretted in so far as their attitude and influence with the medical profession had the effect of causing retardation and submergence of the work for several years."[24]

Despite the opposition in the next few years, a number of encouraging reports followed.[25, 26, 27, 28]

In October, 1929, Dr. George McCoy, director of the Hygienic Laboratory of the United States Public Health Service (later incorporated into the National Research Institute at Bethesda, Maryland), visited the Murdock Foundation Laboratory in New York City where Doctor Glover conducted his researches. In contrast to the investigating committee of the Toronto

Medical Society, Doctor McCoy was favorably impressed. His invitation to Doctor Glover and his associates, Doctors Engle and Clark, to work in a semi official status at the government laboratory in Washington was accepted.

On March 31, 1933, the Public Health Service published a very brief bulletin by Glover and Engle. It reported that a laboratory animal had been inoculated with a virus they claimed to be cancerous and that the virus had been recovered from the animal. This evoked another wave of hostile criticism, "directed not only against the work but those who permitted its publication." [29]

It had been intended that this bulletin be followed by a more extensive report based on work of a greater scale, a project which Doctor McCoy approved. In 1937 Doctor Glover and his associates completed their studies and announced their readiness to publish their findings under government auspices, with Doctor McCoy writing an introduction. In a letter of November 29, 1937, to the Assistant Surgeon General, Doctor McCoy wrote that he still regarded Glover's work as an important approach to the cancer problem, perhaps the most important that had come to his attention in connection with Public Health Service studies while he was administratively concerned with cancer research. The letter was intended as the foreward to the Glover report.

But a subterranean resistance continued to delay publication. The manner in which it worked can be deduced from the following chronicle of events: [29]

A committee was appointed by the Surgeon General to consider the question of publishing the Glover associates' findings. After reviewing their paper, a majority of the committee approved it for publication.

Surgeon General Parran then suggested that a member of the National Advisory Council should also meet with the committee, and a special session was called to permit the presence of this added member. Then, a majority again voted to publish the Glover paper.

The Assistant Surgeon General and the director of the National Institute of Health then suggested that a footnote be added to relieve the Institute of any responsibility for the views expressed, despite the fact that supervision and observation had been invited during the entire course of the work with the Glover microorganisms and Doctor McCoy had signified his willingness to accept the work on the same basis as that of his own research workers.

Instead of a footnote, a statement was incorporated into the paper that constant supervision had been requested but had not been carried out because of the lack of qualified personnel. With this incorporation, the paper was presented and approved for a third time by a majority of the committee. The Surgeon General then ordered Doctor McCoy to write a foreword, which was submitted shortly thereafter. In spite of the annoying delays, everything finally appeared to be settled.

But again a conference was held, attended by all the interested parties. One of the minority committee members who opposed publication suggested that the Glover work should be repeated and confirmed by members of the Institute staff before it was scheduled for printing. The Surgeon General approved this suggestion, thus nullifying previous agreements and cancelling the approval of the committee for publication. Doctor Glover and his associates naturally were confounded, for they felt that such a check should have been arranged at the beginning of their studies instead of after eight years of intensive effort. Since the additional studies proposed would require at least two years more, they refused to wait for publication of their paper under government auspices. Instead, the paper was published in 1938 under the auspices of the Murdock Foundation of New York City.[29] The United States government thereby lost a signal opportunity to sponsor the virus approach to cancer which has become highly respected in recent years despite intense opposition during many previous decades.

In 1940 Glover and White published *The Treatment of Cancer in Man*,[24] based on the treatment of 237 cases of cancer, with follow-ups on 50 patients originally reported in 1926. The malignancies were meticulously described according to site, operability, length under treatment, survival periods and so on. A highly significant rate of recovery was reported. It was also claimed that malignancy could be determined by a blood-serum test devised by Dr. O. C. Gruner of McGill University. Many cancer patients were still alive and well fourteen years after their initial treatment.

Yet these impressive results have never been recognized, in spite of the fact that the work of Doctors Glover, White, Engle and Clark appears to have been a great scientific achievement. In 1955, Stanley of the University of California, was awarded a Nobel prize for identifying a cancer virus; however, no clinical results have followed his discovery.

Doctor Glover is still in practice in Toronto, but he has ignored requests for information on his present work. He is regarded as a very uncommunicative individual, difficult to approach. He no longer publishes his findings; whether this is the result of becoming embittered or he has been effectively silenced is open to question.*

---

* See bottom page 199.

CHAPTER 6

Koch and Glyoxylide

IN THE battles over cancer, the war that raged against Dr. William Frederich Koch is an epic in ruthless ferocity. The discoverer of Glyoxylide, an oxygen catalyst which purportedly increases the capacity of the cell to burn off toxins, is usually referred to by his enemies as the "quack who fled to Brazil to escape prosecution by the Food and Drug Administration." His product is ridiculed as nothing but distilled water.

Doctor Koch's background, however, is hardly that of a charlatan. Born in Detroit in 1885, his degrees are A.B. (1909), M.A. (1910), Ph.D. (1917), all from the University of Michigan; and M.D. (1918), Detroit College of Medicine. From 1910 to 1913 Doctor Koch taught histology and embryology at the University of Michigan, and from 1914 to 1919 he was a professor of physiology at the Detroit Medical College.

Before he was thirty years old, Doctor Koch made a significant scientific contribution to endocrinology by his work on the parathyroid glands. These tiny glands, attached to each side of the thyroid, were once carelessly snipped off by surgeons when they removed goiters. Death from tetany inevitably occurred because the parathyroids regulate calcium metabolism. The *Journal of the AMA* heralded Koch's work in 1913 with a highly laudatory editorial. Six years later, in the same pages he was to be branded as a faker.

In his work on parathyroids, Koch discovered that

removal of the glands brings a marked coagulation of blood and tissues. As cancer patients display the same characteristic, he reasoned that cancer might be due to a toxic condition related to a hormonal deficiency brought on by injury or irritation. This heightened coagulation is a protective mechanism which also stimulates tumor growths. Koch therefore attempted to remove the toxins with tissue thrombin, a ferment which brings on a fever whose heat burns off the toxic elements in the system. This approach was similar to Coley's, but Koch apparently produced curative fevers a little more consistently with tissue thrombin and thereby secured better results.

When Koch boldly claimed a cure for cancer based on the results of treating eight cases,[30] he became a marked man. His claims were derided, and he quickly fell into disfavor with the reigning surgeons in the Wayne County Medical Society.

Doctor Koch approached the cancer problem from the standpoint that the disease is caused by toxins remaining in the blood system. In line with his original interpretation of sugar oxidation as a function to destroy toxins resulting from metabolic processes which he taught at Wayne University from 1914 to 1919, he believed this to be due to insufficient oxidation. He also believed that germs also produce toxins which are incompletely removed, thus subscribing in part to the virus theory of cancer and leading quite naturally to his belief that the solution to the cancer problem lay in securing more active catalysts to stimulate the body's capacity to oxidize toxins.

This reasoning led to the creation of Glyoxylide. According to Koch, his preparation starts a chain reaction in which toxins are converted into antitoxins by the addition of molecules which alter their composition. It was also Koch's belief that the cancer germ or virus is originally harmless but becomes virulent when poisoned by the toxins in the system.

This highly ingenious reasoning, although based on authentic physiology and chemistry' appears a bit too magical. A substance which through some alchemy actually converts a toxin into an antitoxin seems incredible. However, opponents of Koch's theories have formulated no scientific arguments to refute it. Without any investigation, Koch's theories have always been peremptorily dismissed as nonsense.

The Koch treatment does not consist entirely of Glyoxylide but also includes a rigid diet which excludes all foods which are toxic or which contain oxygen inhibitors, such as meats, beans, lentils, coffee, alcohol and tomatoes. Only distilled water is permitted, and daily enemas are prescribed. Neither Glyoxylide alone nor diet alone will cure cancer; according to the Koch school, each must be used in conjunction with the other. One injection of the catalyst is usually effective for six months, and additional injections are not given until decreased oxidation is again evident. The treatment has the advantage of not requiring hospitalization; it is said to greatly alleviate pain, obviate the use of narcotics and stimulate the appetite.

The Koch theory of cancer is as follows: "Clinical observation disclose the persistence of toxemia over a period as long as twenty years previous to the advent of the growth. After the growth has come, these toxic manifestations disappear or nearly so. After a surgical removal of the growth they return and with recurrence of the growth again disappear. We designate these symptoms as the pro-growth symptoms for they differ from those consequent to the activity of the growth itself. The strongest and the sufficient proof that cancer is a response of protection against a definite toxin, however, rests with the fact that removal of the toxin and destruction of the toxic sources is followed by complete involution of all cancer tissue, complete healing of the regions involved, return to health, with absence of growth and pro-growth symptoms, and the absence of recurrence."[31]

In the recovery process, according to the Koch theory, the cancer cell is digested and eliminated by being "split into the chemical elements from which it is constructed, namely, amino acids, fats, sugars, salts, and certain toxic substances. The food materials are turned back to the blood to renourish the body. The toxic substances must also be absorbed but are useless and toxic and they are eliminated through the kidneys, burned up through fever, or passed out in the perspiration, feces and mucous secretions."[32]

Koch's theories strongly contradict prevailing opinion. His internal treatment of cancer, correlated with diet, would relegate surgery and irradiation to the discard. Koch went so far as to say that a surgeon who speaks of curing cancer by operation "not only belies the statistics but he shows his ignorance of the minute structure of the body, together with his ignorance of pathology."[32]

Koch's outspoken criticism put surgeons in the same embarrassing position as the obstetricians, who were accused by Semmelweiss of spreading puerperal fever with their contaminated hands. Surgery and biopsy, Koch said, only spread cancer faster but, unfortunately, surgeons dominated the practice of cancer, had the power to pass on the merits of cancer cures and naturally resented such forceful criticisms. That is the bizarre position into which Koch was thrust, and his subsequent career became a desperate struggle against the interests whom he opposed but who could brand him as a "cancer quack."

The first battle of the "Koch Cancer Cure" war, and one that decided the issue forever in official medical circles, took place in Detroit in 1919. In response to popular pressure, Mayor Couzens, one of the original founders of the Ford Motor Company and later a United States senator, was responsible for initiating a test of the Koch remedy. The procedure devised is one of the fairest and most practical ever proposed in cancer investigations. Unfortunately, its provisions were ignored and nothing conclusive ever came of it.

The plan called for a committee of five examining physicians, appointed by the Wayne County Medical Society, to select the patients for treatment by Doctor Koch and to observe his results. In other words these officials were to be responsible for the selection and diagnosis of patients, and Koch, was to be responsible for their treatment. Certainly nothing could be fairer. There could be no charge against Koch in the matter of selecting patients; that responsibility rested squarely on the shoulders of the committee, none of whom was friendly toward Doctor Koch. According to Koch, this is what happened:

Seven advanced and hopeless cases of internal cancer were selected. They were not local patients, but picked from widely scattered communities and had been brought to Detroit for treatment in a special hospital ward. For three weeks not one member of the committee certified a patient's condition over his signature, the necessary step before Koch could start treatment.

The patients were sinking fast; obviously the greater the delay, the more difficult would be the cure. Aroused, Doctor Koch appealed to the president of the medical society, who whereupon demanded angrily that the committee perform its duty. One patient—and only one—was examined. The diagnosis was hopeless, spreading, internal cancer.

Doctor Koch claims that to avoid criticism he immediately instituted treatment of all patients without waiting for their examinations by committee members. According to Koch's supporters all seven patients responded exceedingly well after only three weeks of treatment. The committee then called the test off alleging that Doctor Koch refused to cooperate, and sent the patients home with a warning not to have anything further to do with Koch.

According to the AMA version of the test, published in its *Journal* of February 12, 1921, Koch was a difficult and uncooperative personality. It was alleged that after the committee went over the cases with him, he demanded permission to name a member of the committee and that permission was granted but that he failed to name his man. It was also alleged that after this meeting Koch gave his injections to the patients but never returned to treat them further. So some patients left in disgust, and the committee sent the rest home.

Here are both sides of the story. More conflicting versions would be difficult to improvise.

Doctor Koch claims that every effort was made to follow up the results of his treatment but that he could trace only three patients. One of them was the patient examined by a member of the committee, as had been agreed upon. Her cancer had originated in the uterus, had spread to the stomach and had caused severe hemorrhaging, but she made a dramatic recovery, according to Koch. Her husband signed an affidavit that her recovery started within three weeks after the injection had been given and progressed to a complete cure. The patient died in an accident fifteen years later. Autopsy disclosed no existing cancer.

A second patient was found to be in good health several years later, free of hemorrhages, pain and the cancerous growth. She testified that as soon as the treatment had been given, her pain had been relieved. The third case that Dr. Koch was able to trace had had an inoperable stomach cancer, with severe pain and hemorrhaging. In 1923 an affidavit certifying to her recovery was submitted to the Wayne County Medical Society in an effort to secure a fair hearing for the Koch treatment.

The hearing was set for November 5, 1923. In the meantime the chairman received a letter dated October 29 from the "Propaganda Department" of the AMA to this effect:[31]

"There appears to be no reason or warrant for a further examination of the 'Koch Cancer Cure.' . . . In spite of the unfavorable report of the Wayne County Medical Society (publicized in its bulletin and in the A.M.A. Journal) . . . Koch has continued to commercialize his alleged cure.

"To take any further action in this case would, in our opinion, simply serve to advertise Koch and give his 'cure' a dignity which is not in the public interest."

Nevertheless, the Cancer Committee of the Wayne County Medical Society did convene. Doctor Koch brought before them a number of patients whose condition had been diagnosed as hopeless by various local physicians but whom he had cured. He also presented patients still under his treatment. The committee denied both the diagnoses and the evidence of cure and, according to Koch supporters, attempted to dissuade patients from further treatment by Koch and to persuade them to undergo surgery instead.

One case which Koch presented was supported by the affidavit of his patient's husband and a witness. They certified that the patient's condition had been diagnosed by a surgeon as Paget's disease and he had advised an immediate operation, as the cancer had spread from her breast to her armpit and clavicle. The patient refused the operation because she was given no assurance that she would retain the full use of her arm.

Instead she turned to the Koch treatment. The surgeon in question was permitted to examine her during the course of her recovery and he eventually acknowledged she had been cured in the presence of her husband. Before the committee, however, he testified that his original diagnosis had been falsified and that the patient's condition had been "a simple ulceration without associated lymph fissuing."[31]

Professor W. A. Dewey of the Department of Medicine at the University of Michigan had been present at the hearings. Writing later to Doctor Koch to congratulate him on the honesty of his presentation before the committee he said of it:

"For a studied intent to falsify, a premeditated determination to condemn everything, and an unscientific, un-American assumption to be judge, jury, and prosecuting witness, the report of this so-called committee outstrips in bias, unfairness, and mendacity anything that has ever been my lot to observe in a medical practice of forty-four years. . . . The composition of the committee, being for the most part surgeons and radium or Xray 'experts,' a class that assumes cancer to be curable only by these methods, was unfortunate in the first place, and in the second place, no member of the committee was, in my opinion, qualified to sit in judgment on your treatment, by education, experience, or by right."[31]

Another of Doctor Koch's friends was Dr. A. R. Mitchell, for many years chairman of the Board of Trustees of the American Medical Association. He wrote Dr. Koch several commendatory letters and advised him, on the strength of his intimate knowledge of the tactics of his confreres, to withhold publication of further information on his cancer preparations or methods. A Detroit girl was alleged to have plied her charms in an unsuccessful attempt to get to the letters away from Koch. Allegations were also made that certain interests closely identified with official medicine tried to gain control of the Koch formula; unable to grab it, they resorted to a campaign of vilification and persecution.

This oppression was extended to those who dared to employ Glyoxylide. It became dangerous for physicians to endorse the Koch method, for they were immediately threatened with loss of their academic and professional standing in the medical profession. These threats were allegedly employed successfully against Dr. Carroll W. Allen, professor of surgery at Tulane University, and against Professior Bryan, head of surgery at Vanderbilt University. Both reported good results but were coerced into discontinuing the use of the Koch preparations.

It is claimed that Professor Maisin of Belgium endorsed the Koch method for some years. Significant support was also found in Canada in the person of Dr. Forbes Godfrey, an eminent Toronto physician who also served for twenty-six years as Minister of Health and Education and who personally visited the Koch clinic in Detroit during his term of office. He extolled the Koch remedy before Parliament as being far superior to radium, of which he said ominously: "Radium has a dangerous effect on the human system. In a couple of years people who have used it usually die suddenly because it affects the heart."

The only cancer investigation with a semblance of dignity and fairness was the in camera sittings of the Cancer Commission of Ontario, Canada, held in 1938, 1939 and 1940 for investigating Glyoxylide. Patients were presented before the commission, which consisted of five members, three of whom were physicians. In many instances, laboratory findings were submitted. The proceedings were conducted in a dignified and impartial manner and elicited many proofs of cure in cancer and other conditions.

A case of endarteritis obliterans (inflammation of the inner coat of the artery) in the foot was presented which had been injected with 1 c. c. of Glyoxylide. Thirty hours later, the black discoloration turned to red; the next day it became pink; ten days later the foot was warm, circulation and full feeling had been restored, and the color was normal.

Dr. H. M. Candlish testified that he had used Glyoxylide on more than one hundred patients in seven months for a wide variety of conditions. Eight cases of coronary disease had responded well, as confirmed by electrocardiograph tracings. Other conditions helped were essential hypertension, eczema, asthma, general debility and cancer. One case had been certified as cancer by biopsy.

The most complete testimony was rendered by the late Dr. J. W. Kannel, a surgeon of Ft. Wayne, Indiana. Before adopting the Koch preparation, he had operated upon at least fifty cases of cancer in his practice, and had followed his surgery with Xray or radium treatment but the longest survival period had been only two and one-half years.

Doctor Kannel testified that he had first learned of Glyoxylide in 1925. He tried it first on a patient with breast cancer who was expected to live only a few months. Instead she survived but suffered a recurrence in 1931. She responded quickly to additional treatment and was reported as alive and well in 1939.

In 14 years, Doctor Kannel attested, he had treated 72 cases with the Koch preparation. Many of these he considered hopeless to treat but he was forced to yield to their insistent pleadings. He reported that 21 of his cancer patients were still alive at the time and that four had died of other causes. Some of these survivors had traveled to Canada to testify.

Doctor Kannel also mentioned the professional hazards involved in adopting the Koch treatment. A colleague had been expelled for his local society merely because he "talked too much about it." Yet Glyoxylide was the only remedy that had offered him hope in treating cancer, Doctor Kannel said, in contrast to his poor results prior to 1925, after 24 years of operating for cancer.

On a visit to the Mayo Clinic, he also mentioned seeing a surgeon remove five cancerous breasts in one day. When he asked if surgery, followed by Xray and radium would cure the cancer, the surgeon admitted great pessimism but said he knew of nothing else to employ.

In spite of impressive evidence offered at the Canadian hearings, no formal findings were ever published. To prevent the Koch adherents from capitalizing upon them, the chairman of the Canadian Cancer Committee stated in the July 19, 1941 issue of the *Journal* of the AMA: "It should be noted that this commission has made no report expressing any opinion whatever of the efficicacy or otherwise of the Koch treatment as a remedy or cure for cancer."

In 1940 and 1941 Doctor Koch conducted work in Mexico and Brazil on leprosy, tuberculosis and mental conditions. He claims to have brought about a rapid cure of dementia with one injection of Glyoxylide. This reputedly so incensed a representative of a big pharmaceutical firm then reaping huge profits from useless drugs injected repeatedly into mental patients. He is reputed to have shaken his fist in Doctor Koch's face and warned him that he would not be interfering much longer in Brazil.[31]

In April, 1942, Doctor Koch was arrested in Florida on a charge that his product was falsely labeled. At the hearing, $10,000 bail was asked. The Federal Commissioner demanded an explanation for this unusual request; such bail is customary only in murder cases. The district attorney then disclosed that he had been ordered from Detroit to insist on the high bail to prevent Doctor Koch from returning to Brazil and finishing his researches there.

In 1942 and 1946, the United States Food and Drug Administration prosecuted Koch in two bitterly fought trials. The government attacked the oxidation theory of curing cancer and contended that, according to the opinion of their experts, the remedies were indistinguishable from distilled water. A temporary injunction against the Koch Laboratory was granted pending a thorough Federal Trade Commission hearing. The injunction was made permanent in 1950.

Utterly exhausted and defeated, Doctor Koch gave up, relinquishing his methods to the Christian Medical Research League of Detroit. This organization then inherited the Koch formula and was called upon occasionally to defend physicians threatened with malpractice proceedings, expulsion from medical societies or loss of their medical licenses because of using Glyoxylide.

In 1952 a physician in the Middle West was expelled from his local medical society for "unethical" practices —the use of Glyoxylide. Local newspapers published letters from grateful patients. One former patient told reporters that she had been cured of cancer by the expelled physician after having been given only a few months to live following surgery and Xray treatment by another doctor. Her cancer disappeared after two injections costing only $50. "They were certainly worth it," the woman commented. "I had spent $1,300 before that."

In 1954, Dr. C. E. Hardy of Nashville, Tennessee, was brought before the medical examiners and deprived of his medical license. He had prescribed the Koch treatment and found it successful in a number of cases. No patients had complained against him, some testified for him, but he lost his license.

The powerful punitive measures that can be brought against physicians using an outlawed remedy, regardless of whether the proscription is justified or not, is a deterrent against independence of thought. It has proven effective in finally destroying Glyoxylide and putting it off the market. As of this writing, it is no longer manufactured. It is said that after Koch gave up the battle and assigned his manufacturing process to a Detroit religious organization, the preparation was incompetently processed and was no longer effective.

The career of William Koch who now lives in Brazil, is indeed a tragedy. If his theories are scientifically unsound, they can be scientifically demolished. If his clinical claims were false, a fair test would disprove them. Instead, Koch was driven out of practice by the concerted and relentless prosecution of medical societies and government bodies. The Koch case proves once again that no scientific standards for testing cancer exist and that the fate of an independent cancer therapist, regardless of his scientific training and qualifications, is inevitably the same. The competent and incompetent alike, the quack and the dedicated healer, the fraudulent and the genuine are damned equally, without the slightest attempt to award them a fair hearing.

CHAPTER 7

The Hoxsey Saga

$\mathbf{A}$T THE California cancer quackery hearings, the shadow of a powerfully built man with a lantern-like jaw hovered over the proceedings. It was the shadow of Harry M. Hoxsey, the tough, crafty, dogged, truculent individual who has been the bane of the American Medical Association for almost forty years and vilified by his enemies as the worst cancer quack in history. According to Benedict FitzGerald, the Washington attorney who has represented Hoxsey in several legal battles, he is the most dramatic, colorful and impressive personality in the cancer wars.

In the life-and-death struggle Hoxsey has waged with the AMA, he has been fined, jailed and prosecuted more times than any other man in the history of cancer. He has fought back tooth and nail; matched his cunning and ruthless opponents with equal cunning, craft and resourcefulness; and used every influence and force he could muster in his dog-eat-dog struggle. In the fight, Hoxsey has not been too meticulous in his choice of allies, several of whom were pretty unsavory characters. Among others were Norman Baker, the notorious quack, and Gerald Winrod, the anti Semitic demagogue, publisher of *The Defender*.

Yet at the same time, Hoxsey will brazenly boast of his Jewish friends, some of whom edited and published the absorbing saga of his struggles.[33] On the cover jacket, under the portrait of "Harry M. Hoxsey, N.D.," reads this informative bit of biographical data, typical of his flamboyant showmanship:

"I am 54 years young.* For 35 of those years I have
been kicked, hounded, persecuted and prosecuted because I've treated cancer with medicine and without
the use of surgery, Xray or radium.

"As the poet says, I've stood 'like a beaten anvil'
on the theory that the more they beat, the louder the
noise; the louder the noise, the bigger the audience;
and the bigger the audience, the sooner the truth shall
be known.

"This is my story."

And a grotesque yet fascinating story it is, a genuine
piece of Americana. Even the obvious touching up of
the facts, the self-glorification and the profuse sprinkling of half-truths and propaganda in the book, does
not detract from its interest. I expected to meet something of an idealist with a flair for showmanship, so
cleverly is Hoxsey's case pleaded in his book.

But after talking to him on intimate terms in his
office in Dallas, my conception became more realistic.
I found him talkative to the point of garrulity, though
he was also extremely shrewed, and a man who can
drive a hard bargain. His talk is down to earth and
sprinkled so liberally with SOB's and other profanities
it smacks of the gutter. Hoxsey is primarily for Hoxsey and the saga of his struggles is tinctured with his
yen for lucre. Nor has he done badly.

From the original source of his fortune in cancer
therapy, he is reputed to have extended his investments
to oil, real estate and other endeavors. His newest enterprise is the promotion of virus-free eggs. Hoxsey
claims that most cancer patients are heavy egg eaters
and eggs are produced in an unsanitary manner which

* Hoxsey was born October 23, 1901.

loads them with viruses. These viruses, he contends, cause not only cancer but a host of other diseases. His "Bonded Egg" venture is a result of his forced withdrawal from cancer practice as he now can only rent his clinic which no longer carrys his name.

Hoxsey prefers to be addressed as "Doctor." His degree is "N.D." I did not inquire whether he was a naprapath or naturopath, nor how he attained it. In all probability, it is a "mail order" degree. In his account of his career, he makes no mention of any formal studies. Because he has been surrounded by cancer almost all his life, Hoxsey's practical knowledge and experience are far superior to anything taught from books or in a school. He claims to have assisted his father in his cancer practice from the tender age of eight. He learned to apply dressings, talked with patients and naturally had innumerable opportunities to observe the manifestations and progress of the disease.

Evidently he learned well for his school was life itself and his teacher was his "daddy" whom he quotes constantly for his astounding wisdom. Whether this reverence is genuine or just good hokum, like so many other of Hoxsey's characteristics, is problematical.

Hoxsey's extraordinary stamina and toughness which carried him through the long and grueling fight with the AMA is a result of his boyhood lot. Reared on a farm, Hoxsey became acquainted early with back breaking toil. As the family was large and the income from the farm and his father's combined veterinary and cancer practice was meager, Hoxsey had to work in the coal mines near his birthplace in southern Illinois.

Soon he became a mule driver in the mines. According to his story, he was fired with the ambition to become a doctor and was on the lookout for every chance to make an "honest dollar." He drove a cab, too. This was particularly lucrative on pay days when the miners flocked to brothels in neighboring towns.

Hoxsey also boasts of his athletic prowess. He claims to have pitched for a professional baseball team and attained such fame, that a major league baseball team "scouted" him. He also professes to have engaged in professional boxing and to have mixed with no less a fighter than Jack Dempsey. Since Hoxsey has a touch of the Baron Munchausen in him, some of his vainglorious boastings border on the psychopathological.

The Hoxsey saga begins in 1840 on the Illinois farm of Harry's great-grandfather, who owned a valuable Percheron. The animal had a hopeless cancer on his right hoof, according to a veterinarian, who suggested he be destroyed. Instead, the doomed horse was given free rein on the Hoxsey pasture.

But the horse miraculously recovered and his tumor sloughed away. As the animal showed a special fondness for one corner of the pasture, his choice of fodder was carefully noted. According to the family legend, John Hoxsey ground up various combinations of the plants the Percheron selected and found a remedy for cancer in farm animals. He prepared a liquid, a salve and a powder and kept his formula secret, attaining a considerable reputation as a veterinarian through his concoction.

Therefore like Plunkett's of the seventeenth century, the Hoxsey remedy was family property but it also had the unusual distinction of originating with an animal, if the Percheron story is true. The remedy would then be a product of the animal instinct for survival, developed millions of years before man. The feeding instinct of animals and their acceptance or rejection of foods has long been celebrated as uncanny. That aspect of the Hoxsey history is therefore credible.

As the years passed, the Hoxsey remedy was used in human cancer. In the family tradition, Harry Hoxsey's father prepared his own liquids, salves and powders on his farm and brought a year's supply to his office in town. Harry began to "like" cancer and was fascinated with his father's work. His keen interest in cancer delighted his father though Harry was the only child in their large brood so inclined. As there are indications that his father's meddling in human cancer was resented by physicians, Harry in all probability also inherited his father's feud with them.

In 1919, Dr. John Hoxsey contracted erysipelas. On his death bed, he summoned Harry, his favorite son, and ordered him to bring his safe deposit box together with three tablets of writing paper. When these were brought, the dying man dramatically asked his son to close his bedroom door and come close. Sitting up with great difficulty, he fumbled among his papers, brought out a small white envelope and then solemnly said:

"These are the cancer formulas I got from my father and he got from his. Now it's my turn to pass them on. I have twelve children and I love you all the same. But when you were just a little shaver, asking questions about my work and watching me treat patients, I knew you had the call to be a doctor."

With his dying breath, the man praised his son's industry, his fortitude and thirst for knowledge. Because of these qualities though the youngest of his children, he alone was selected to inherit the precious formula. But Harry was commanded to write out the formula for the liquid over and over until he filled every page in one of the three tablets. The task took many hours; Harry Hoxsey claims he fell asleep while writing and finished the next morning.

When the completed copying was brought to him, the elder Hoxsey carefully burned the original and copies, certain then his son had indelibly committed the precious formulas to his memory. The same ceremony was repeated with the salve and powder formulas.

"Now you have the power to heal the sick and save lives," Harry Hoxsey's father solemnly said. He implored his son to bring the boon of their remedy all over the country and all over the world; to cure tens of thousands where he had cured hundreds. He bound his son by a sacred oath to be faithful to his trust and never lose touch with the "common people", nor to refuse treatment to those who could not pay. He also warned him dolefully of the fierce enmity of the medical profession because he would be taking money out of their pockets by curing cancer.

"They're powerful; they're the High Priests of Medicine," the dying man warned, "But in the end you'll win. Because there's one thing they can't do, and that's put back the cancer you removed."[33]

Then he died and Harry Hoxsey became sole proprietor of the family remedy at the age of eighteen. Though determined never to use it until he was a qualified medical physician, Hoxsey claims the cure was too well known and he was sought out and implored for help. His first patient was a Civil War veteran who was pledged to secrecy but after he was dramatically cured, told others who also besieged Hoxsey for help.

His successes became known in Chicago, where Hoxsey was invited to demonstrate at a clinic. Dr. Bruce Miller, a staff member, became so impressed that he consented to become medical director of Hoxsey's cancer clinic at Taylorville, Illinois. Doctor Miller was evidently a man of some competence and loyalty for he was associated with Hoxsey during some of his most trying periods. He later moved to Los Angeles where he treated cancer with escharotics with some success for a number of years. He is still living but very feeble because of his advanced age. I was able to locate Doctor Miller in Los Angeles but he was not in a condition to talk, even over the telephone.

(As a sidelight on Hoxsey's character, in mentioning Doctor Miller I observed that he must have been a wonderful teacher. Hoxsey replied, without a trace of gratitude, "He learned from me too.")

With Doctor Miller as director, the Taylorville Clinic was supported by the local chamber of commerce and was very successful for a time but a fateful incident soon brought on the long and bitter war between Hoxsey and the AMA. This transpired when one of Hoxsey's friends was able to arrange a demonstration of his therapy to be sponsored by Dr. Malcolm Harris, a renowned Chicago surgeon who was secretary of the AMA at the time. Later he became its president.

It was agreed that Hoxsey and Doctor Miller would be allowed to treat a hopelessly afflicted cancer patient at Chicago's Alexian Brothers Hospital. Thomas Mannix, a police sergeant with advanced cancer of the clavicle was the patient. He was sadly emaciated according to Hoxsey, badly burned by repeated Xray treatments and emitted the typical odor of rotting flesh. Though Doctor Miller despaired, Hoxsey claims he was not dismayed and began treatment with the utmost confidence of a cure.

The recovery was miraculous. The patient was displayed before the entire hospital staff and Doctor Harris professed his utmost amazement and delight. Hoxsey was jubilant, though Doctor Miller was skeptical. When Doctor Harris summoned Hoxsey to his office

very early the next morning, he thought he was on
his way to a brilliant future under the most respectable and impressive medical auspices.

At their meeting, Doctor Harris reputedly said:

"Hoxsey, the demonstration you put on yesterday
has opened up an entirely new vista in the treatment
of cancer. I spent most of last evening discussing the
Mannix case with some of my colleagues and they agree
that his amazing recovery is convincing evidence that
chemical compounds such as you use offer the best hope
to eradicate the disease."

Hoxsey could scarcely restrain his giddy sense of
triumph and an "impulse to jump up and gratefully
shake his hand."

Doctor Harris however, cautioned him against over
confidence as it was premature to pronounce a cure;
five years without a recurrence must pass before claim-
ing recovery. He also wished to test the remedy on
many other patients. When Hoxsey eagerly volunteered to show him hundreds of patients already cured,
Harris said a more scientific proof was needed. Large
scale experiments under medical controls which would
select certified cancer cases would have to be set up,
he maintained, and the patients kept under strict supervision to rule out other factors which could contribute
to recovery or relapse. It was a long range project
which would require careful planning.

When Hoxsey assured him of his cooperation, Doctor Harris quickly produced a legal contract which he
said had been prepared in advance, because he was
confident Hoxsey would be cooperative. It was ten
pages long and demanded the surrender of the Hoxsey
formula to Doctor Harris and his associates; the relinquishing of all claims in their favor; the delivery of
ample supplies of the internal medicine, powder and

ointment and the instruction of their representative in mixing the compounds. Hoxsey was also to close his clinic and give up treating cancer forever. After a ten year experimental period, he was to be paid 10 per cent of the net profits thereafter.

Stunned after reading this "incredible document," Hoxsey relates he read it again to be sure he had understood correctly. Shocked by the harsh terms, he feebly asked for time to consult the family attorney. His powerful adversary snapped back that no changes would be tolerated in the contract; those conditions were final and no others would be considered. Unless the contract was signed, Hoxsey was told he could not see Sergeant Mannix again. Orders to that effect were phoned at once to the hospital. Hoxsey's narration then reads:

"I waited until he hung up the receiver, then seized the telephone and called the Mannix home. Before I could be connected, Doctor Harris reached over the desk and tried to take the telephone away from me. My left elbow flipped up, caught him squarely in the chest, and sent him flying into his chair. It promptly toppled him over, depositing him in a most undignified position on the floor."

Hoxsey then instructed the patient's daughter, a registered nurse, to get her father out of the hospital as he would change his dressings at their home. Livid with rage, Doctor Harris picked himself off the floor and shrieked he would have Hoxsey jailed if he treated Mannix again. He threatened to have his clinic closed and run "that quack doctor of yours out of Illinois."

So began the Hoxsey-AMA cancer feud. It was long and bitterly fought and only a man of Hoxsey's iron constitution could have withstood the relentless warfare. The Taylorville clinic was immediately attacked.

Hoxsey confesses that his own sisters and brothers were hoodwinked into suing him for a share in the profits of the family formula. Hoxsey succeeded in defeating their suit but he lost his clinic.

In the stormy years that followed, between intervals at Detroit and in West Virginia, Hoxsey was associated for five months with the notorious Norman Baker of Muscatine, Iowa. There he broadcast over Baker's radio station and no doubt learned the art of propaganda, showmanship and the need for cultivating powerful connections. However Hoxsey and Baker could not get along; the latter was too greedy he said, to say nothing of his lechery.

In speaking of his Muscatine experiences, Hoxsey related a lurid tale of a gun battle. According to his tale, he was "tipped off" over the long distance telephone by a man with a decided Italian accent that three gunmen were leaving Chicago to "knock you off." The caller described the men and their car minutely. Hoxsey believed the mysterious caller was friendly because he had once cured the cancer of the mother of a notorious gangster. When the gunmen arrived, they were driven off by a hail of bullets, so he said.

In 1936, Hoxsey established himself in Dallas, Texas where he won some measure of affluence by developing strong political and business connections through the gratitude of cured cancer patients. However, the increase in his cancer practice was always attended by law suits, injunctions, arrests for practicing medicine without a license and continual brushes with Fishbein. The highlight of his legal battles was a slander suit won against both Morris Fishbein (his first such loss) and the Hearst newspapers. The slander was a statement that Hoxsey's father had died of cancer but it was proved that he had succumbed to erysipelas.

In another momentous case, a federal judge ruled that Hoxsey sometimes cured cancer, that patients were helped in many cases and that the testimony of patients in reference to their own cancers was admissible legal evidence. This decision was temporarily Hoxsey's greatest legal victory. Later a higher court overruled it.

In 1954 a Hoxsey clinic was opened in Portage, Pennsylvania, which touched off the usual controversy. Hoxsey was associated in this venture with a former state senator John J. Haluska, a somewhat bombastic and flamboyant figure. Once administrator of the Miner's Hospital in Johnstown, Pennsylvania, he had been removed after a bitter battle with the physicians on the staff.

In an interview, Haluska related he had become intensely interested in cancer because of the toll the disease had taken in his own family. His mother and several close relatives had been victims but the most tragic death was that of his only child, a boy of nine born with a tumor behind his ear. For years physicians who were his friends advised him against an operation for the boy.

One day however, it was suggested that a renowned Philadelphia specialist could easily remove the boy's tumor which was becoming embarrassing. Haluska took his boy to Philadelphia and despite his terror and his pleas to his father not to permit an operation, it was performed. The boy expired on the operating table.

In 1953, Senator Haluska's sister, a mother of four children, was stricken with an inoperable cancer pronounced hopeless by various experts. She was flown to Hoxsey and allegedly cured. When Haluska then attempted to introduce the Hoxsey therapy at the Miner's Hospital, the entire staff threatened to resign unless he was ousted.

Haluska resigned and under a partnership agreement with Hoxsey, several business men and physicians who comprised their staff, a Hoxsey Cancer Clinic was established in Portage, Pennsylvania. The first year of operation was financially successful, according to figures presented by the government in a suit to close the clinic.

No verdict was rendered at the first of such trials, but at a second in the fall of 1957 both parties agreed to a consent decree. The clinic thereby refrained from using literature or making claims of a cancer cure, agreed to properly label its medications and to prescribe them according to usual medical procedures. In turn, the government dropped charges and the clinic is still in operation, although recent reports indicate that measures are again being instituted to close it. Hoxsey displays but little interest in the clinic, and intimated that he now holds a low opinion of the Senator.

At this writing, Hoxsey can no longer practice in Texas because naturopathy has become outlawed. He has leased his clinic to an osteopathic physician, who operates under his own name. The clinic still finds it extremely difficult to secure staff physicians because they are threatened with a loss of their license for associating in the Hoxsey treatment.

Just what value the treatment has is still very difficult to ascertain. The only remotely impartial or scientific investigation was undertaken by Doctor Ivy, who for the first time publicly admitted visiting the clinic at the San Francisco hearings. Doctor Ivy was somewhat dubious about the Hoxsey treatment in internal cancer and attributed its action in external cancers to potassium. This again confirms the opinion of the English physician Forbes Ross who, before the turn of the century, said that every so-called quack remedy could always be found to contain potassium.

At the San Francisco hearings, the spokesman for the National Cancer Institute testified that the seventy seven cases the Hoxsey Clinic had submitted were rejected as inadmissible because no pathological data were included. According to Hoxsey, the cases submitted were either confirmed by biopsies or the Institute was informed where biopsies could be secured. Here again are two conflicting statements over matters of fact by opposing interests.

The Hoxsey cancer saga consequently embodies all the usual features of every cancer controversy. It includes the refusal to examine so-called cured patients, ceaseless condemnation and opposition, alleged attempts to seize control of the remedy without compensation or credit, and endless litigation compounded of intrigue, corruption and suppression of evidence. The personality of Hoxsey himself, however, has given his particular story a unique aspect as his own tactics and his own motives are not irreproachable.

At last he has been forced to withdraw from further treatment of cancer personally. He has finally been defeated, although he did manage to amass a fortune. At this writing, attempts are still being made to carry on his work both in Texas and California (the status of the Portage Clinic is in doubt). Whether these attempts will succeed without benefit of Hoxsey's tremendous drive, audacity and resourcefulness is quite doubtful. If the Hoxsey clinics eventually are closed, the last chapter will have been written in the most unusual and fantastic story in the history of cancer, if not in the history of healing.

CHAPTER 8

Three Independents

GREGORY'S ANTIBIOTICS

For some years, Dr. John E. Gregory of Pasadena, California, has devoted himself to the hypothesis that cancer is virus-caused and has presented his views in a well-illustrated monograph.[34] The introduction states that the study represents "the result of exhaustive and careful research work, all of which has been repeated by competent men in their fields. The research outlined here has cost the author over $250,000. It is the result of more than 20,000 hours of research in the field of cancer. In the past ten years, forty weeks have been spent at research clinics and at scientific meetings which pertained to this subject."

In another passage Doctor Gregory states that he wishes to erase any impression that the employment of "essential or early surgery and radiation can be neglected in the treatment of cancer. Rather it is the author's hope that all pharmaceutical laboratories and all research laboratories will be inspired to a more active program in the search for additional antibiotics which may be effective in the treatment of cancer."

In his research, Doctor Gregory employs an electronic microscope in magnifications as high as 50,000. On the basis of animal experiments, he defines cancer as "an infectious disease in which the infecting organism is a cancer virus, which sensitizes cells to grow invasively and metastasize, when stimulated by chemicals, irritants, or excess hormones. An overwhelming infection may produce the disease."

Doctor Gregory claims that the cancer virus develops an enzyme which he identifies as chymotrypsin. In an effort to determine whether the cancer virus is a product or a cause of the disease, he performed laboratory experiments to fulfill Koch's Postulate. These experiments required that the injection of a culture from malignant melanoma into laboratory animals be followed by the recovery of the virus from the malignancy which developed in the test animal. When this virus is proved to be the same as the one injected, it presumably fulfills Koch's criteria, and Doctor Gregory claims to have completed this test successfully over fifty times.

If cancer is virus-caused, then the treatment of choice is antibiotics. The difficulties in their use are resulting toxic reactions and the fact that strains of viruses will develop an immunity to antibiotics, which then lose their effectiveness. Antibiotics have greater value in acute infections; in chronic diseases the bacteria gradually develop resistant strains. To overcome this difficulty, according to Doctor Gregory, many different antibiotics will have to be used to offset the different resistances that develop in the course of treatment.

In his attempts to develop a suitable cancer antibiotic, Doctor Gregory isolated from the white mold of the streptomyces family, an antibiotic which he called "Gregomycin." He claims that it is nontoxic, that it brought tumor regression in animals and that in clinical tests 80 per cent of the patients improved when given this antibiotic daily by injection and 20 per cent did exceptionally well.

In clinical investigations begun early in 1952 with more than one hundred far-advanced cancer patients, Doctor Gregory claims to have discovered an even more effective antibiotic, Antivin. He reported that patients treated with Antivin experienced immediate improvement in appetite and decrease of pain. The results were so encouraging that all other antibiotics were abandoned in favor of Antivin.

The clinical results claimed are improvement in 80 per cent of the patients treated, and entire regression of tumors in 20 per cent, with continued good health. The diet recommended is free of meat and fat but contains enough calories to prevent loss of weight. A high fruit diet is also advocated.

This summarizes Dr. John E. Gregory's independent researches and clinical results. His work is interesting and commendable because it was wholly independent and was financed entirely from his own resources—expenditures reached over $250,000. In view of the tremendous amount of time, money and effort expended by Doctor Gregory, his efforts are entitled to the highest respect and considerations. Unfortunately, they have been appreciated only in a very limited circle. Doctor Gregory has met the usual haughty and peremptory rejection by the authoritarian bodies, and his work has not been investigated officially, despite the fact that it is based on researches and conclusions published in orthodox cancer journals. There is a question, of course, whether or not Doctor Gregory's claims and conclusions are justified, but that could be determined only by a fair and scientific investigation. To this observer, his presentation appears somewhat amateurish and his reasoning somewhat arbitrary. But any person who has invested the time and effort which Doctor Gregory has expended deserves a fair investigation. There appears to be nothing harmful in his ministrations, and his antibiotic has been carefully checked for toxic effects. His results appear to compare favorably with those of other methods of cancer therapy.

THE LINCOLN BACTERIOPHAGES

One of the darkest palls in the history of cancer therapies, has enveloped the work of the late Dr. Robert E. Lincoln of Medford, Massachusetts. The manner in which the blackout was effected also provides one of the most illuminating examples of how the dominating interests work together and can discredit an independent physician despite his excellent approach and noteworthy results.

Lincoln was a physician of excellent qualifications. He began to study medicine after his discharge from service in World War I, entering practice in 1926. In addition to his practice, he engaged in research in supersonic energy as applied to medicine under the direction of Professor George W. Pierce of the Laboratory of Applied Physics at Harvard. Doctor Lincoln also invented a mechanical heart pump during this period.

Later, while still in general practice, Doctor Lincoln became fascinated by the problems of virus diseases which were bringing a new and changing pattern to the incidence and prevalence of many afflictions. In a paper announcing his discoveries which was read by Ernest Mills, M.D., at a meeting of the Medford Medical Society on December 12, 1951, this is how he described the unfolding of his work:

"I noted in all my patients suffering from acute or chronic frontal sinus infections, and also in those with no evidence whatsoever of sinus headaches, that over 90 per cent had been ill at some time in the past with one or both of the two types of 'epidemic grippe' that have been repeatedly recurring over the previous 35 years in a rapid and steadily increasing volume. Over 85 of every 100 patients who have been at some previous time infected with the causative germs of these two infectious and contagious ailments would never again be completely free."

In endeavoring to discover the cause of the tremendous increase in sinus infections, Doctor Lincoln cultured various germs he found in the sinus passages of his patients. He succeeded in isolating two pure strains of the most malignant and poisonous germs in existence, and designated them as Hemolytic Staphylococcus Aureus (Lincolnii), Alpha and Beta. These germs, he reported, were hosts for the perpetuation and multiplication of two distinct and related viruses which he also isolated the Alpha virus on June 5, 1946, and the Beta virus on November 24, 1946. Of these, Doctor Lincoln wrote:

"Both host cells or germs are capable of destroying the red blood cells, or damaging any particular tissue in the body by a process of toxic congestion; or of causing abscess formations, which may be single, or so numerous as to join together and cause partial or total destruction of either the working or the structural tissue of any organ, or of both types of tissue . . . Each host germ has one, and only one, particular strain of virus as a partner. These viruses use their respective germ as a refuge in which to live and grow when they are not in contact with and destroying the specific body tissue cells which they prefer, just as all disease-causing germs and viruses show a marked choice for certain specific tissues."

Doctor Lincoln's therapy was to inject at regular 48 hour intervals solutions containing the virus, which had the capacity to seek out the host cells and destroy them. He believed this would occur under natural and normal physiological conditions in "the nasal passage, nature's own bacteriophage chambers" if it were not for anatomic obstructions offered by old swollen mucous membrane surfaces and old strains of weak host cells, which in turn completely control and thereby weaken the in-partner viruses.

Doctor Lincoln claimed that the Alpha germs were capable of metamorphosing into a Beta strain and that the Alpha virus could not only destroy its host, but the Beta germ as well, while the Beta virus did not have this reciprocal relationship.

Doctor Lincoln correlated various flare-ups and epidemics with marked changes in weather, and observed that an exceptionally severe drop in his weather-quotient statistics brought on a marked change in symptoms. He attributed this to the metamorphosis of the Alpha to the Beta host cells.

In treating his sinus cases, Doctor Lincoln secured approximately 95 per cent "apparent cures." Where there were secondary conditions such as arthritis, angina, deafness, blindness or some forms of degenerative disease, these conditions decreased and disappeared at the same rate as the sinus condition. In cases which proved recalcitrant, it was necessary to administer the Beta virus, which led to the treatment of many chronic conditions in which there was no sinus infection. In describing this phase of his work, Doctor Lincoln stated:

"As treatment of patients with a variety of illnesses progressed, it became increasingly evident that an answer had been found for the hundreds of perplexing disease symptoms or groups of symptoms plaguing humankind today, such as a never-ending feeling of tiredness, chronic dizziness, leg-muscle cramps, mental depression, sudden maniacal outbursts, as well as other abnormal forms of human conduct, together with the more frequently occurring sudden destruction of large numbers of red blood cells, forming embolae.

"With the continued passing of time, the number of 'incurable' diseases capable of being 'apparently cured' has continued to increase until they include practically the entire list of disease conditions for which no known cause or cure exists. This includes cancer."

The inclusion of that last taboo-ridden disease caused Doctor Lincoln to become involved in the typical chain of events attending a new cancer therapy. First of all, he was besieged by patients. His fees ranged from $1.00 to $5.00 and no one was turned away. The Lincoln Foundation, a charitable and nonprofit institution, was organized to distribute his remedy.

One of Doctor Lincoln's most famous cancer patients was Charles W. Tobey, Jr., son of the late senator from New Hampshire. Mr. Tobey made a dramatic recovery and was so interested in Doctor Lincoln's work that he became active in extending its benefits to the world at large. He soon learned that there was a deep and decided aversion to acknowledging the Lincoln discoveries. Every avenue of recognition suddenly and mysteriously became closed, until in April, 1952 Doctor Lincoln was expelled from the Medford Medical Society for his caustic criticism of his colleagues.

Senator Tobey became so incensed over the blackout of Doctor Lincoln's work that he presented a bill of particulars to his colleagues in the Senate on February 11, 1952, itemizing in detail the various snubs and rebuffs meted out to the physician. The following are just a few:

In the fall of 1946, the *Journal of the AMA* summarily rejected Lincoln's paper on his clinical results with his antibiotics.

In January, 1948, the same paper was submitted to the *New England Journal of Medicine*. In August,

1948, it was rejected for "lack of space." But as Senator Tobey pointed out, space was found for "The Vitamin D Content of Mare's Milk."

In March, 1948, Doctor Lincoln wrote to a large Boston hospital inviting a research commission to study his work. The director wrote that he was "unable to find the time" for such a project.

Three letters to an editor on the staff of the *New England Journal of Medicine,* requesting assistance in arranging publication of the work by Doctor Lincoln, were ignored.

In October, 1948, Doctor Lincoln requested to no avail, a leading popular magazine to assign one of its writers to observe his work.

In 1949, Doctor Lincoln requested conferences with leaders of the Massachusetts Medical Society. Tentative meetings were scheduled but were repeatedly postponed. Although the Society had never investigated the Lincoln therapy, its letters advised inquirers that the treatment was of no avail.

In August, 1949, the president of the American Medical Association declined to render any assistance in securing a review of the Lincoln work. In his estimation, the difficulty was a "local one" which he thought Doctor Lincoln must solve.

After Senator Tobey had inserted his son's letter in the *Congressional Record,* describing his dramatic cure and that of several other patients, he was deluged by letters from cancer sufferers. He advised them that assistance would be rendered provided their physicians visited the Lincoln Clinic. After a number of physicians from various parts of the country did visit the clinic to examine case histories and Xrays and to interview patients, some of them became interested in serving as research fellows in the Lincoln Foundation and in administering the antibiotics in their practice.

According to Senator Tobey, because of the demand to investigate the therapy, the Massachusetts Medical Society reluctantly appointed a study committee. It had first tried, however, to refer the matter to a committee on ethics and had circulated a derogatory press release aimed at belittling the Lincoln discoveries.

Doctor Lincoln then called at the offices of the society to insist upon the appointment of the study committee. The society complied, but limited the committee to surgeons.

In August, 1951, the committee interviewed several patients on the back porch of Doctor Lincoln's home. The following month, it did the same. The committee then agreed to a request for a hospital study, but in the ensuing months absolutely nothing was done to fulfill this obligation despite repeated reminders, nor has it ever been completed.

Then something happened which revealed the malignant nature of the influences behind the opposition to Doctor Lincoln's work. A letter from the dean of the Boston University Medical School, in whose laboratories the Lincoln antibiotics were always prepared, notified the Foundation that its supply had been cut off. The director of the laboratory had been forbidden to deliver any of the antibiotics already prepared.

This stoppage was maintained for fourteen days. In one hospital, 75 patients had to go from seven to ten days without medication. It required the pressure of urgent telegrams from members of Congress to induce the dean of the Boston University Medical School to resume supplying the antibiotics until another laboratory could be set up to take over the work.

When, after six weeks, the university laboratory did turn over the cultures to the newly created laboratory for the Lincoln Foundation, the original strain was not present in the cultures, another piece of skulduggery. Had it not been for the fact that Doctor Lincoln had maintained cultures of the germs in various places, production would have been completely sabotaged.

On March 6, 1952, after eight months of so-called study, the medical society finally issued its report. It was the standard rejection, incorporating all the old familiar arguments that have not changed and which can be written without examining any evidence whatsoever.

The report discredited the cure of Senator Tobey's son because the surgery and Xray treatment he had undergone before taking the Lincoln treatment might have been responsible. Remember, the committee was composed chiefly of surgeons; internists or bacteriologists were not included. The committee's contention that "equally beneficial results from Xray and surgical treatment in this disease have been reported on patients who did not receive Doctor Lincoln's treatment" is therefore quite consistent with the policy of maintaining the *status quo* of surgery and Xray as the treatments "of choice." The report concluded with the statement that in the committee's "honest and considered opinion, based on all the available evidence, no proof has been presented, nor was any able to be obtained, which has shown that beneficial organic changes have occurred in disease processes treated by Doctor Lincoln's therapy which have been due to that therapy and to that alone."

Doctor Lincoln characterized the report as "in keeping with the past high degree of stupidity that has been maintained by this segment of the American Medical Association." The Massachusetts Medical society thereupon requested his resignation. When it was not forthcoming, Doctor Lincoln was expelled on April 8,

1952. He died in January, 1954.

The loss to the public of an inexpensive, effective and salutary cure for many chronic conditions is incalculable. In contrast to the derogatory opinion of the study committee of the Massachusetts Medical Society is the report of May, 1957, from a prominent physician of the state, quoted by Senator Tobey in his address in the Senate:

"The 65 severe, chronic cases which I have treated were selected because of their severity and longevity. All of them have been completely relieved, with the exception of two patients. I feel that I now have a non-toxic bactericidal agent with which I am able to effect complete relief, both subjectively and objectively."

It is significant that the physician's name was not disclosed. Unquestionably, a report of this nature based on treating many severe and chronic cases, over an extended period, is of real medical and scientific authenticity. The report of the Massachusetts Medical Society was based on three visits to Doctor Lincoln's clinic and on interviews with patients on the back porch of his home.

Yet when Senator Tobey wrote to more than one hundred medical schools, requesting them to send representatives to the Lincoln Clinic to investigate and study the therapy, he was told that such a study was being conducted by the Massachusetts Medical Society and that it would be unethical for them to enter the picture.

As was testified at the California hearings, the National Research Council and other government institutes involved in cancer work closely with the American Cancer Society, the American Medical Association and other influential bodies. The extent of this close association and its method of operation can be discerned from Senator Tobey's investigation of the reception accorded to the Lincoln therapy by government institutions.

After receiving numerous appeals from veterans considered hopelessly afflicted with cancer and tuberculosis but who grasped at the hope of the Lincoln treatment, on October 8, 1951, Senator Tobey requested the Veterans Administration to investigate the Lincoln therapy. On the following November 30, the medical director of the Veterans Administration replied that the National Research Council had advised against making any such investigation. The report of the Massachusetts Medical Society had not yet been rendered, presumably because not enough patients had been interviewed on Doctor Lincoln's back porch, so the refusal was undoubtedly based on a "tip" as to what the findings of that society's "investigation" would be. The hands-off policy toward investigating the Lincoln therapy, as evinced by medical schools, hospital clinics and medical journals and also maintained by government affiliated institutions, therefore gave the Massachusetts Medical Society, on behalf of the AMA, the sole and final say on the value of the Lincoln treatment.

Senator Tobey became impatient at the run-around. He protested directly to Doctor Rubey, chairman of the National Research Council, and threatened to lay the facts before members of Congress and the public. He pointed out that research groups throughout the country had refrained from investigating the Lincoln therapy because they were under the impression that the National Research Council was to undertake the study, whereas Doctor Rubey had advised that it would not do so because the Massachusetts Medical Society was to conduct the investigation. The senator demanded an explanation for Doctor Rubey's statement that the council was in close touch with the society's investigation, in view of the fact that the Massachusetts Medical Society actually had done very little.

Tobey declared that the council was not living up to its responsibility in protecting the health of veterans and the public, and demanded a showdown. A meeting of interested parties, which included Doctor Boone of the Veterans Administration, and Drs. Rubey and Winternitz of the National Research Council, was held in his office on January 8, 1952. Charles Tobey, Jr., was present to testify to his own cure by the Lincoln method. Numerous letters from tuberculous and cancer-ridden veterans requesting the VA to investigate the Lincoln therapy were also read.

Doctor Winternitz (who, it will be remembered, reported on the basis of the AMA "status report" that Krebiozen was worthless) was asked why members of the National Research Council in the vicinity of the Lincoln Clinic had not made their own investigation. He replied that representatives were not sent to investigate a new therapy until a formal request had been received.

Senator Tobey confronted Winternitz with the written proof that such a request had been made by the acting Surgeon General of the United States Public Health Service on December 20, 1951, nineteen days prior to the present "showdown" meeting. A second letter was produced, also written on December 20, 1951, and addressed to Senator Smith of New Jersey by the National Cancer Institute, advising that the National Research Council had already been requested to evaluate Doctor Lincoln's method. Whereupon Winternitz went into a huff and threatened to leave the room.

A veteran afflicted with Hodgkin's disease then presented proof that the medical director of the New England division of the Veterans Administration had approved a course of Lincoln treatments for Hodgkin's disease patients but that no action had been taken. At this disconcerting evidence, Doctor Boone, the director of the VA, then pulled a "Russian withdrawal" and without further ado departed with Winternitz and Rubey.

Their strategy was obvious. The men apparently knew that the report of the Massachusetts Medical Society was foreordained to doom the Lincoln therapy. The public was highly aroused over the Lincoln investigation incident, and the atmosphere created by Senator Tobey was decidedly unfavorable for the publication of an unfavorable report. So they simply stalled, hoping that public indignation would ebb and that the Massachusetts Medical Society could issue its "findings" without rearousing public indignation.

Their trick worked. The report was published in March, 1952, and Doctor Lincoln's expulsion from the medical society followed.

Senator Tobey's summary to his colleagues, written about a month before the status reports of the medical society was published, concluded:

"The foregoing demonstrates forcibly the obstacles that are placed in the path of one who has devoted his life to medical research and to the alleviation of human suffering."

Those obstacles are the same ones that every independent worker in medical research, particularly in cancer, has always had to face and has never been able to surmount. Despite its inherent promise, the Lincoln therapy is today virtually unknown. Its use is fraught with the hazards of ostracism and expulsion that attend physicians who minister Glyoxylide, Krebiozen, and other controversial therapies.

THE BEARD-KREBS APPROACH

Another theory of the origin of cancer—the unitarian or trophoblastic thesis—is sponsored by the John Beard Memorial Foundation of San Francisco, which is directed by Ernst T. Krebs, a physician, and Ernst T. Krebs, Jr., a biochemist. The originator of this concept, John Beard, D.Sc. (1858-1924), eminent in comparative embryology and vertebrate morphology, spent almost his entire career, from 1890 to 1921, in the Department of Natural History of Edinburgh University.

On the basis of Beard's studies of the embryology and morphology of vertebrates, he announced in the *Lancet* of June 1902 a theory of cancer which can be summarized briefly:

Embryos develop a distinct type of cell, the trophoblast, which appears immediately after fertilization and exercises a special function—eroding a site in the uterine cavity for the growing foetus. This power of erosion is contributed to the genesis of the embryo, just as other types of cells contribute the unique properties determined by various genes.

Because of their destructive power, the continued active existence of the trophoblasts constitute a danger to the embryo once they have served their purpose. At that time (56 days after conception), the foetal pancreas begins to secrete the enzymes trypsin and amylopsin to destroy the dangerous and henceforth unnecessary trophoblasts. Beard contended that if the foetal pancreas fails to function in time and the trophoblasts multiply unchecked, the most malignant form of cancer known—chorio-epithelioma of pregnancy—would destroy both mother and foetus.

According to the Beard theory, the trophoblastic cell and the cancer cell are identical in nature; both have the power to erode, absorb and destroy other cells. When this power is unregulated, it is abnormal and a menace to life.

The clinical application of Beard's theory, first attempted in 1904 by injecting the pancreatic ferments trypsin and its complement amylopsin, failed. It is now contended, this failure was due to the lack of adequate control over the chemical composition of the ferments produced at that time by pharmaceutical firms or individual clinicians.

Beard wrote that his approach was opposed because of the "intolerance" (in human nature) of the new and strange, even though this be calculated to be of surpassing benefit to humanity.

"Sooner or later," he said, "it will be recognized that, while the ferments of cancer came into existence in the dim and distant past for the purpose of building up asexual generation, trypsin and its complement, amylopsin, were evolved millions of years ago as things even more powerful . . . and for the primary purpose of pulling down the asexual generation. . . . If the enzyme treatment of cancer be abandoned for the next century (nevertheless) every human being who comes into the world . . . will never fail . . . to use the pancreatic or enzyme treatment of cancer in his own gestation for the suppression of normal trophoblast or asexual generation (lest) this, as the most deadly form of cancer known—choreoepithelioma—would inevitably destroy him and his parent."[35]

The Beard Foundation contends that after a study of 17,000 papers on cancer and its pathology, forty-

three common and identical characteristics of the trophoblast cell and the cancer cell have been found, without disovering any points of dissimilarity and that the
trophoblastic concept therefore constitutes an all-em-
bracing theory of cancer based on biological and pathological observations which have never been disproved.

Currently, the therapeutic application of the Beard
trophoblastic theory is worked with Laetrile, an enzymatic substance derived from the apricot kernel. Experiments with this substance were begun in the 1920's
by Dr. Ernst J. Krebs, in the hours he could spare from
a large medical practice and were financed from his
personal income.

Doctor Krebs inherited his interest in pharmacology,
toxicology and herbal substances from his father, a
well-known pharmacist of before the turn of the century, who insisted on preparing his own extracts from
plants and herbs. In World War I, Doctor Krebs
achieved international fame in halting the influenza
epidemic in the vicinity of Carson City, Nevada, with
the use of the sacred herb of a local Indian tribe which
he discovered gave them immunity to colds and infections.

In the 1920's, Doctor Krebs concluded that the
proper enzyme or ferment would dissolve the protein
of the cancer cell. From the glucoside-rich kernel of
the apricot, he extracted an enzyme which he believed
could accomplish that feat. On applying it to animals
afflicted with spontaneous cancer, he met enough success to encourage a trial with human cancer. Although
some patients responded, the preparation was toxic and
could be administered only as a last resort.

It is claimed, that in 1952, Krebs, Jr., analyzed his
father's preparation and concluded its cyanogenetic
properties accounted for the destruction of cancer cells.

He separated the enzyme Emulsin from these cyanogenetic substances, and it is claimed that when these
substances were administered separately at short intervals, the toxic hazards to the cancer patient were
eliminated.

Laetrile, according to its proponents, substantiates
the Beard trophoblastic theory by authenticating a
common denominator in cancer and trophoblastic cells
—high concentrations of the enzyme Betaglucoronidase.
This enzyme is vulnerable to the very deadly hydro-
cyanic gas. Laetrile purportedly gives off this gas when
combined experimentally with suitable ferments and
therefore cures by lethally gassing cancer cells.

This peculiarity of the cancer cell is believed due to
its deficiency of Rhodanese, the enzyme which is a normal component of healthy tissues and dispels hydro-
cyanic gas when it forms in the system after the ingestion of certain foods. According to its discoverers,
Laetrile therefore destroys cancer cells without harming the Rhodanese-protected normal tissue and has a
highly selective action.

Three principal methods of administering Laetrile
and its auxiliary, Beta-glucosidase, are used:

1. Parenterally—injecting the preparation into the
muscle in the case of inaccessible internal cancers.

2. By tamponade—soaking the preparation in cot-
ton and applying it directly to the malignant area.

3. By iontophoresis—pushing the preparation in solution directly into the tumor by means of an electric
current. This method is used in breast cancers and
other accessible malignant growths.

Dietary recommendations require abstinence from
all milk and dairy products, which require chymotrypsin for digestion. This pancreatic enzyme also has anti-
carcinogenic properties. When dairy products are

eliminated from the diet, this enzyme is free to work against cancer. A diet of fruits and vegetables is recommended; nuts are also approved except in cases of stomach and bowel cancer.

On the whole, Laetrile therapy is claimed to be painless, to avoid damage to normal tissues and the need for narcotics. Though Laetrile has not been recognized or become generally known in the United States, some physicians in Italy and the Philippines have claimed some encouraging clinical results with it. However, these reports do not contain very convincing proof, and little is known about current therapy with Laetrile in this country due to the timidity of its proponents for advancing their claims or to their lack of impressive results.

CHAPTER 9

Two Lay Remedies

THE DROSNES-LAZENBY TEAM & MUCORHICIN

AT THE San Francisco hearings, the inability of Dr. Joseph Wilson to testify concerning the Drosnes-Lazenby Clinic because of his scheduled tour of Navy duty prevented disclosure of one of the most fantastic stories in the annals of cancer. It is a tale of two amateurs—a former tire dealer and a hospital dining room supervisor—who pooled their talents in a search for a cancer remedy. Their search culminated in the substratum (the liquid exuding from a mold processed with whole wheat, yeast and distilled water) which they labeled "Mucorhicin."

They have stirred up considerable interest in their preparation for the treatment of cancer and allied diseases, including arthritis, peptic ulcer and some skin disorders A considerable following of patients and friends have become their sponsors and have battled valiantly in their cause. In the course of their controversy and struggle to secure recognition, the Drosnes-Lazenby team have received national though unfavorable publicity; have been arrested for practicing medicine without a license and acquitted of the charge, and have had their remedy administered to thousands of patients with some very interesting results.

The Drosnes-Lazenby collaboration with the assistance of Dr. Paul Murray, (Doctor Wilson's predecessor as medical director) is a fantastic tale. On the surface it is hardly credible that a man with absolutely no scientific or medical background and a woman with only a modest experience as a hospital employee could discover an authentic cancer remedy. Yet tests on animals and on human cancer patients have proved that Mucorhicin has definite biological action. Drosnes and Lazenby therefore have succeeded without bothering to formulate complicated hypotheses or arguments or to secure grants, and without elaborate scientific apparatus. Their approach was simple and direct because they are two simple and direct people. This is how it all came about:

In 1944, Phil Drosnes and Mrs. Lillian Lazenby met socially. They chatted about medicine, and Drosnes exchanged a little bandinage with the woman about the ignorance of doctors.

"See, I am bald-headed," he told her, "but what do doctors know about growing hair? I am also somewhat deaf, but what can they do about improving hearing? Nothing. What do they know about curing cancer? Also nothing."

Mrs. Lazenby then confided that she was intensely interested in finding a cure for cancer as she had always had a terrible horror of the disease because her mother had died of it after intense suffering. Drosnes displayed interest; a favorite uncle of his had died from the same malady. He agreed to help in her search for a cancer cure.

Their unique partnership was born. As blithely as if the matter were no more serious than making up a menu or starting a tire-selling campaign, without bothering to collect a Nobel prize or to enlist the aid of biochemists, pathologists or physicians, they embarked on a project to cure a disease as dreaded as leprosy, upon which untold millions had been spent for research; of which hundreds of thousands die every year; and which is the subject of countless medical papers, bitter controversies and constant propaganda. In short, the Drosness-Lazenby team started to solve the mystery of a disease which reputedly baffles some of the greatest minds in the world and which supposedly requires endless years of research and study in biochemistry, physiology, pharmaceutics and practically every branch of medicine in order even to partially understand.

If the discovery of these two average citizens with hardly any of these qualifications is only partially valid, the Drosnes-Lazenby partnership has made a mockery of science. If two amateur physicists had brought about nuclear fission in their kitchen before Fermi did at the University of Chicago, their feat would have been no less astounding. The success of the Drosnes-Lazenby team may signify that:

1. The problem of cancer is not as baffling and monumental as it is dramatized and that its endless complications and mysteries are pure ballyhoo.

2. Cancer is indeed one of the world's most difficult problems but, through some incredible chance impossible to duplicate in a million years, Drosnes and Lazenby succeeded where thousands of the most qualified research workers failed.

3. There are many approaches to the cure of cancer, and many different biochemical substances, readily available to everyone can be valuable in cancer therapy.

The last may be the most likely possibility.

Mrs. Lazenby started her search with a very valuable clue. In 1944 there was a great fanfare about penicillin and the work of Fleming and Waksman in antibiotics. She undoubtedly heard about their work and may have learned something about it from the discussions of physicians in her hospital dining room. The approach in which she interested Drosnes was based on the discoveries of brilliant men and was therefore on solid ground.

The Pittsburgh couple toiled in the basement of her home with the crudest of materials and facilities until they found what they wanted—an enzymatic product derived from processed whole wheat grain. In the course of her experiments, Mrs. Lazenby also came to believe that she could detect a cancer parasite in the blood stream.

This again is a highly controversial subject, but the woman either had immense self-confidence or a naivete beyond calculation. Lacking even a microscope or funds with which to buy one, she and Drosnes were forced to borrow an instrument whose magnification power Drosnes still does not know. With this microscope, Mrs. Lazenby claimed she could detect a cancer virus and devised a test to locate it in the blood stream. This blood test was later to involve them in many difficulties and to arouse great derision. Like the method of producing Mucorhicin, the blood test became a closely guarded secret but it is no longer advanced and was discreetly relegated to oblivion.

After processing Mucorhicin, in the approved fashion, cancerous guinea pigs were secured for testing with it. Results were encouraging. The next step was to try it on human beings. Three hospitalized cancer cases, pronounced hopeless, were fed Mucorhicin in their orange juice without their knowledge. This is a "blind test" with a vengeance; certainly no psychic influence could be present. According to Mr. Drosnes, the three patients showed marked alleviation of symptoms and a return of appetite and energy, but the disease was not arrested and they died.

Later, Drosnes and Mrs. Lazenby were permitted to treat hopeless cancer patients who had been discharged from hospitals to die at home. The two drove to the homes of these hopeless patients twice a day to administer their extract. There were some dramatic, if only temporary, remissions and even some cures among these terminal cases. When it was no longer possible to take care of their widely scattered patients, advice was sought in April, 1948, from John H. Teeter, then a director of the American Cancer Society. He suggested that a clinic be set up in Pittsburgh under medical direction; and according to Drosnes, if results proved interesting, he promised financial assistance.

Under the medical direction of Dr. Paul A. Murray, a Pittsburgh nose and throat specialist, a clinic was set up in the basement of a Catholic church. It was as fortunate as it was unusual for a licensed medical physician to risk his professional prestige to espouse a remedy discovered by laymen, but Doctor Murray was an unusual man. As a medical student at the University of Pittsburgh, he had led his classes in scholarship every year, something never accomplished before or since. About a year later after the clinic was established, Dr. Joseph Wilson joined Doctor Murray as an associate. He became director of the clinic when Doctor Murray died in 1954 of a cerebral hemorrhage brought on, it is believed, by overwork.

Just after the establishment of the Drosnes-Lazenby Clinic, which was directed in accordance with the American Cancer Society's suggestions, the troubles of the two began. In October, 1948, Drosnes and Mrs. Lazenby were arrested for practicing medicine without a license and were convicted. The conviction was set aside and a new trial was ordered, but the case was dismissed because it was easily proved that the clinic had been under medical direction.

The case created quite a stir of publicity, and the

opposition took notice. A newspaper reporter, representing himself as a cancer patient recommended by a physician had a sample of his blood taken at a hospital and sent to the clinic. There it was diagnosed by the Lazenby test as cancerous, according to the newspaper man. Later it was discovered that chemicals had been added to the blood specimen to give it a false reaction. Since that time, the claim for the Lazenby cancer test has been withdrawn, very probably because it cannot be substantiated and exposes its originator to just such machinations. The reporter then described his hoax in sensational stories, which became the basis for allegations of quackery by medically affiliated organizations.

The DrosnesLazenby Clinic, however, had staunch friends among the patients who had been helped and among their friends and relatives. Treatment had often been given free and these humanitarian efforts were not unappreciated. The tactics employed to ridicule and discredit the DrosnesLazenby team leaves the distinct impression of cheap skulduggery and chicanery regardless of the merits of their claims. The fact that the medical profession or the organizations believed to stand for a scientific approach to a medical problem utilized a newspaper man's hoax and could not refute the claims of two laymen by authentic, scientific methods indicates that no such methods exist or that the opponents are ignorant of a truly scientific method of disproving false claims. All through the DrosnesLazenby dispute, this impression remains quite strong, because the very lack of scientific qualifications by the discoverers of Mucorhicin would appear to make them vulnerable to a purely scientific refutation.

The publicity attending their trial increased the furor, and the Pittsburgh City Council demanded an investigation. Dr. R. R. Spencer, reputedly the real life inspiration for the hero of *The Green Light,* the novel by Lloyd Douglas, came from Washington in his capacity as an adviser in behalf of the National Cancer Institute. His presence was requested by I. H. Alexander, director of the Pittsburgh Health Department, in response to popular demand.

Two conferences were held by Doctor Spencer with interested parties. These included Mr. Drosnes and Mrs. Lazenby; Doctor Murray, their medical director; officers of the Allegheny Medical Society, the American Cancer Society and the University of Pittsburgh; and Doctor Alexander, director of the Health Department. Doctor Spencer suggested a plan of certifying the results of treatment and outlined the requirements of the National Advisory Cancer Council, then left for Washington. He is alleged to have promised to return in six months to advise further, but he never did. The Drosnes-Lazenby Clinic also charged that his plan was pigeon-holed and that the minutes of the meeting were suppressed and never made public.

Opponents of the clinic, however, alleged that the conference constituted an "investigation" of the Drosnes-Lazenby claims, which were found fraudulent. The principal disseminator of this allegation was the director of the City Health Department.

The same state of confusion exists in regard to a chemical analysis of Mucorhicin. A sample of the mold was sent to the National Cancer Institute and the mycologist rendered a report in which he stated that he had identified various forms of antibiotics (principally Rhizopus and Mucor, from which Mucorhicin derives its name) and also excrement, spores and "scales of unidentified insects."

This report was distorted by opponents, who alleged that the substrate itself contained these impurities.

When the extract itself was sent to the laboratories of the National Health Institute, however, they declined to analyze it because of the lack of qualified personnel and because they believed it would be of little value. The Institute suggested that only clinical tests could establish the value of Mucorhicin. Samples sent to the Council on Pharmacy of the AMA also evoked the excuse that facilities for making a chemical analysis did not exist.

That summarizes the "testing" of Mucorhicin. Yet on such flimsy data did Walter Winchell allege that the Drosnes-Lazenby Clinic had been found guilty of quackery, and the editors of the now defunct *Colliers* brand the discoverers of Mucorhicin as cancer quacks.

Nevertheless, Dr. J. W. Wilson, director of the Drosnes-Lazenby Clinic, can point with gratification to a number of successful cures. Many of his patients, once dismissed by other physicians as incurable, are still living. In the ten years since the clinic was established, it claims to have treated over 3,000 patients through dispensing physicians without any reports of toxic reactions or untoward effects. The proportion of symptomatic relief, "such as alleviation of pain, eating, sleeping, and feeling better before death," has been more than 90 per cent of all cases.

So almost two centuries after Richard Guy, a member of the London corporate of surgeons adopted the controversial remedy of the Plunkett family, the Doctors Murray and Wilson of Pittsburgh similarly renounce the measures employed by their colleagues in the treatment of cancer and advocate a remedy developed by two amateur biochemists.

THE HERBS OF REES EVANS

The ramifications in cancer controversies are truly

surprising. One of the most bizarre involves Rees
Evans, of London, inheritor of a cancer remedy originated about 1905 by his father and uncle in Cardigan,
Wales. After their herbal preparation had cured an
older brother of cancer, it was administered to ailing
friends and neighbors. Highly devout and simple men,
the Evans brothers opened their treatments with a
prayer, imploring the Lord's guidance. In 1907 they
were the subject of two scathing articles in the *British
Medical Journal.*

The unusual feature of the Evans therapy is that although disdained by the English medical profession,
through a curious chain of circumstances it was tested
in the United States under the highly respectable medical cooperation of the Presbyterian Hospital of Newark, New Jersey. No publicity was permitted in the
United States, but *Picture Post,* a popular English magazine now defunct, in 1950, gave the Rees Evans work
here some startling publicity. As a result, the Minister
of Health was obliged to appoint a committee to investigate the Evans method.

Rees Evans had been treating cancer since 1919,
when he returned from war service. His inherited herbal
treatment was soon attacked by the orthodox medical
interests. In 1924 he requested an investigation
and a committee was appointed. Asked for the names
of 20 of his cancer patients, Evans submitted 30. The
committee subsequently reported that it was unable to
locate any of the patients for the purpose of investigating their cures. Rees Evans contended that the
committee had made no attempt to locate these patients,
a number of whom had reported to him that the addresses supplied were correct or that forwarding addresses were available.

In 1930, two experts from the Royal Cancer Hospital investigated the Evans therapy by examining two of his patients but without permitting Evans' presence during their examinations. One patient immediately discontinued treatment with Evans after the examintion and brought suit against him. The trial was long and expensive. A publicspirited journalist, Hannen Swaffer, assumed the costs of the trial which ended in a disagreement.

In 1950, Swaffer summarized his experiences with Evans in a letter published in *Picture Post* on September 23, 1950, in which he cited a number of cures by Evans that he had investigated himself. One was that of a woman Swaffer had referred to Evans after she had been treated at various cancer hospitals with little benefit. A physician who was familiar with her case pronounced her "miraculously" cured after the Evans treatment, and promised to testify in Evans' behalf. But when he was urgently needed at the 1930 trial it was impossible to locate him.

This is the description of a typical Evans treatment:[36]

The patient discovered a growth shortly after suffering a blow on her breast. Following unsatisfactory treatment by a cancer specialist, she consulted Evans. Holding out hope for a cure in about twelve weeks, with a soft brush he applied his solution, which brought sensations of penetration, burning and pulling. The treatment was given six days each week and was painless. The growth gradually drew up until it became hard and black and raised over the level of the skin. A lettuce leaf placed over the tumor turned black. After twelve weeks of treatment the roots of the cancer came away, leaving a crater underneath which was treated by another solution. This too healed, leaving only a small scar.

The patient related that she showed her healed breast to the specialist she had first consulted. "Miraculous!" he too exclaimed, but denied that she had ever had the very cancer that he himself had diagnosed.

When he was invited to the United States in 1950, Rees Evans claimed to have treated about one thousand cancer patients. His invitation came about through somewhat odd circumstances. Mrs. Evans had been in this country to attend a convention and had met Mrs. Ann Lupo of Newark, New Jersey, a woman very active in social work. Mrs. Evans mentioned her husband's excellent results in cancer and his lack of recognition. Mrs. Lupo became interested and was influential in securing an invitation from the Presbyterian Hospital, Newark, to demonstrate his treatment. When Evans arrived, a clinic and sixteen patients were assigned to him. He worked for eight months without compensation, and was at length compelled to return to England to resume practice. He arranged for publication of his American results with *Picture Post* of London.

The Evans article appeared in the magazine on September 9, 1950. Preceded by a dramatic exposition of the gravity of cancer and the inevitable controversies surrounding revolutionary treatments, it was gruesomely illustrated and daringly supplied the patients' names. According to *Picture Post,* the sixteen cases Evans treated were always under strict medical supervision, and all but one (patient 8) had been diagnosed by "the most exact and unquestionable methods known to science and medicine."

The following are the results of the Evans treatment at the Presbyterian Hospital, Newark, New Jersey (from November, 1949, to May, 1950), as published in *Picture Post:*

Patient	Sex	Age	Previous Treatment	Site of Lesion	Duration of Treatment
No. 1	Male	20s	(not given)	Leg	8 weeks
No. 2*	Female	64	Operation	Breast	8 months
No. 3†	Female	44	Operation	Cervical gland	8 months
No. 4	Male	56	Colostomy	Rectum (metas.)	8 months irregular
No. 5	Male	60	(not given)	Larynx	22 weeks
No. 6	Female	44	Hysterectomy complete	Metastases to genitals and liver	9 days
No. 7	Male	40s	Inoperable	Carotid area	22 days
No. 8	Female	72	(not given)	Rectal	15½ weeks
No. 9	Female	89	(not given)	Face	8 weeks
No. 10	Female	50	Arm, thigh, breast (amputation advised)	Breast	8 months
No. 11	Male	88	Excision	Jaw	12 weeks
No. 12	Female	55	None; neglected	Breast	7 months
No. 13	Female	50s	Xray and surgery	Carotid gland	8 months (treatment continued by hospital)
No. 14	Male	55	Much Xray; some surgery	Glands of neck	10 days
No. 15	Male	72	Colostomy 1947	Sigmoid	7 weeks
No. 16	Female	50	Sulpha drugs	Breast	1 month

Compilation of results:

    9 completely cured—including 1 patient who died of pneumonia.
    1 partially cured; treatment continued by hospital.
    1 partially cured; attendance irregular.
    1 failure (internal cancer).
    4 died.

Of these sixteen cases, ten had been regarded as hopeless. Considering that there were nine positive in-

---

* Evans reported this patient as still living but in March, 1958, I could not locate her.

† Patient was interviewed in March, 1958 and reported she was very well.

dications of cure, and that the treatment had been comparatively painless and inexpensive and had not required hospitalization, the results were commendable indeed.

Publication of these results brought a flood of letters to *Picture Post*. Those from physicians were for the most part condemnatory, but few signed their names. All seemed to overlook the fact that the diagnoses had been made according to accepted medical procedures and that the treatments had been under the close observation of the medical staff of the Presbyterian Hospital.

The *British Medical Journal* published a severely critical editorial, which *Picture Post* very effectively reprinted in its September 30 issue, alongside the reply in an adjoining column to each criticism raised. According to the *British Medical Journal,* the Tumor Therapy Committee of the Presbyterian Hospital had cabled:

"Work entirely experimental. No definitive results obtained. Evans' statement unwarranted and unauthorized. No results to be published. Would disavow all unproved claims by Evans."

According to *Picture Post,* however, the American committee had, as late as July 31, 1950, still been interested in continuing the Evans experimental treatment, although it is certain that the Presbyterian Hospital subsequently became "miffed" by the publicity in England. But Mr. Evans was under no obligation to the hospital because he had in no way been compensated for his great expenditure of time and effort and certainly was within his rights in securing publication wherever he chose.

This effective airing of the Evans controversy with the British medical profession prompted the official in quiry that *Picture Post* had hoped to bring about. Aneurin Bevan, British Minister of Health at the time, notified Mr. Evans that an investigative committee had been appointed.

Evans agreed to cooperate, but reiterated in a letter that his work could not be "fully and finally tested unless actual treatment of patients forms part of the investigation." Without examining a patient at the inception of treatment and without observing each result during the course of treatment, the proper investigation of a cancer remedy is of course well-nigh impossible. In view of the psychological factors present, even the method of administration and the physician's professional manner have an important bearing on results.

Yet the distinguished committee took cognizance of none of these factors. Its investigation consisted solely of examining records and of discussing them with Rees Evans and Derek W. Morley, the science writer who had collaborated in the *Picture Post* articles. Its findings, easily predictable and in the usual vein, as reported in *Picture Post* of June 14, 1952, were as follows:

"The committee examined the histories of British and American patients treated by Mr. Rees Evans, and also investigated the materials used by him in his work, as well as receiving oral and written evidence from him. It did not examine patients under treatment since it considered that in most forms of cancer assessment of the results of treatment it is not possible until treatment has ended, and also since the technical details of applying any particular treatment are irrelevant to the assessment of its value in treating cancer.

"Examination of the histories of 22 British patients treated by Mr. Rees Evans between 1931 and 1945 who could be traced from 34 names supplied led the committee to the following conclusions:

Insufficient information for diagnosis................. 5
No convincing evidence of cancer at the time
    of treatment 3
Judged not to have suffered from cancer.......... 7
Death from or seriously ill from recurrence
    after treatment 2
Rodent ulcer 5
    Total 22

"Enquiries were not pursued in the cases of rodent ulcer on the grounds that it is a form of skin cancer of slight malignancy; that it has been known for many decades that it can be successfully treated by several methods which remove the locally affected tissue; and that evidence of success in healing rodent ulcers throws no light on whether the same method will be useful in the treatment of cancers in general.

"Examination of the histories of the American cases treated by Mr. Evans in 1949 and 1950 was also made, and the condition of these patients in July 1951 was as follows:

Dead from cancer... 8
Seriously ill from cancer.................................... 1
No convincing evidence of cancer.................... 2
Condition doubtful 1
No recurrence, but also treated surgically or
    with Xrays 2
Rodent ulcer 2
    Total 16

"Samples of the materials used by Mr. Rees Evans in treatment were analyzed and were tested in experiments on animals. The committee was advised by the leading experts that the results obtained did not provide any indication for recommending further experiments."

Members of the investigating committee were:
    Sir Robert Robinson, O.M., F.R.S., Chairman
        (President of the Royal Society)
    Sir Alexander Fleming, F.R.S.. etc.
        (Discoverer of penicillin)
    Sir Ernest Rock Carling, M.B. M.S., etc.
        (Chairman of the Standing Advisory Commit-
        tee on Cancer and Radio-therapy)
    Professor Himsworth
        (Secretary of the Medical Research Council)
The committee held eight meetings. Mr. Evans was allowed to be present at only two of them. In his absence, unnamed medical practitioners testified on the Evans treatment, and their statements were accepted without the opportunity for Evans to hear or challenge them. On numerous occasions Mr. Evans offered to demonstrate his methods in the presence of the committee but his offers were declined. Evans also questioned the elimination of his rodent ulcer cases and cited the opinion of Willis, one of the leading cancer specialists of England, who regarded rodent ulcers seriously. Willis described their progress as "slowly invasive and destructive. Untreated growths on the face may eventually destroy most of the soft tissues and bones and may penetrate to the skull or the brain."

In general, the report of the committee held that the Evans patients who died did indeed die of cancer, while those who lived either had had no cancer or had been helped by the delayed effects of previous Xray or surgical treatment. This bias is particularly evident in the summary of the American cases, ten of which had had previous surgery or Xray. That treatment was not acknowledged, however, except in the two cases where the patients survived.

The investigation of the Evans therapy discloses that

England does not have any worthier method of inquiry than does the United States and that no really scientific method of evaluation exists in either country. Considering that Evans is a layman, unversed in science or medicine, the distinguished scientists on the investigating committee should have been able to refute his therapy. Yet they resorted to the old familiar prejudiced arguments based solely on authoritive opinions, completely ignoring favorable evidence and considering only unfavorable indications.

CHAPTER 10

New York Schools

THE GERSON THERAPY

In 1946, Senator Claude Pepper of Florida introduced a bill "to mobilize at some convenient place in the United States an adequate number of the world's outstanding experts and to coordinate and utilize their services in a supreme endeavor to discover means of curing and preventing cancer."

Hearings on the bill were held July 1, 2 and 3, 1946, before a Senate subcommittee presided over by Senator Pepper himself. Among those testifying was Dr. Max Gerson of New York City, who appeared with some of his cured cancer patients, several colleagues and a number of supporters. Senator Pepper's bill was subsequently defeated.

At the time Doctor Gerson testified, he was on the staff of the Gotham Hospital of New York. Today he is not on the staff of any hospital. Once he instructed his associates in his method of cancer therapy. Today he finds it impossible to secure medical assistants. Approaching the age of eighty, he now practices alone. For over thirty years he has demonstrated excellent results in treating cancer, his approach is on a highly scientific level, and his credentials are the finest. Yet he has never received a penny to aid in his researches.

The 1946 hearings supply excellent insight into Doctor Gerson's therapy. First to appear on the doctor's behalf was S. A. Markel, of Richmond, Virginia, who testified that the Gerson therapy had cured his osteoarthritis after other physicians had pronounced his case hopeless. He mentioned the antipathy directed toward Doctor Gerson and the accusations of fakery which were used to discredit his claims, even though his clinical results had never been checked.

"I would hate to think that the antipathy to Doctor Gerson," testified Mr. Markel, "would be in any manner associated with the fact that his treatments are dietary and are not surgical. . . . Doctor Gerson has no doubt made enemies as the result of his dietary therapy, wherein he does not permit patients to smoke or drink or to consume canned goods and other items which could materially affect trade."

When Doctor Gerson took the stand, he supplied the following biographical information: He was born in Germany on October 18, 1881. He graduated from the University of Freiburg in 1907 and was trained by such famous internists, neurologists and endocrinologists as Professors Fraenkel, Kroenig, Foerster, Sauerbruch and Zondek, each of whom he served as an associate for varying lengths of time. He has practiced in New York City since 1938 and has written numerous medical articles on cancer research, diet in cancer, and metabolism in cancer.

Doctor Gerson testified that he had developed his dietary approach many years before to relieve his own migraine and then had applied it successfully in asthma and other allergies, in diseases of the intestinal tract, liver and pancreas, in tuberculosis, arthritis, heart disease, skin conditions and so on. His most striking results were obtained in liver and gall-bladder diseases.

Doctor Gerson began treating cancer by diet in 1928. Of his first twelve cases, seven responded favorably, remaining symptom-free for seven and one-half years. In New York City he treated 90 per cent of his patients at the Gotham Hospital without charge and financed his own researches in chronic diseases. He testified that he believed the liver to hold the key to the cure of cancer and that if the liver was too far gone, treatment was useless. The Gerson theory of cancer was placed on file with the Senate subcommittee in the form of a paper, "Case Histories of Ten Cancer Patients, Clinical Observations, Theoretical Considerations and Summary."

Several cured patients were then presented. The first, a teen-age girl was diagnosed with "a cervical and upper thoracic intramedullary glioma." After an exploratory operation at the Neurological Institute of Columbia University, surgeons told her father that her condition would soon prove fatal.

When brought to Gerson, her case was diagnosed as "a paresis in the lower right arm; the process involved especially the nervous ulnaris of the right hand and the right leg; she could not walk much." The growing tumor was destroying her spinal cord so that stimuli could not be carried to the muscles, which were therefore atrophying.

Doctor Gerson testified that his treatment had killed the tumor and that the girl was recovering the use of her muscles. He claimed that this was the first arrest of such a tumor in two thousand years of medical science. This case can be identified as No. 7, in A Cancer Therapy,[37] a work published to supplement and extend Doctor Gerson's 1946 testimony.

To bring her history up to date: The patient was able to type, dance and skate with little or no evidence of any previous neurological disease until 1952, when she began to experience various nervous disturbances. Treatment was resumed and in July, 1957, the patient reported that she had recovered except for stiffness and weakness in her right arm and leg.

The next case presented was that of an ex-soldier, discharged from the army with a diagnosis of "basal cell carcinoma at the back of the right neck, of hair follicle origin and precursor of rodent ulcer." Xray treatments had been regarded as too dangerous; an operation undertaken under the assurance that it would be trivial had resulted in the man's inability to move his head and the formation of a rapidly growing tumor. A second operation was refused.

The patient was brought to Doctor Gerson in extreme pain, attended by dizziness, loss of equilibrium, swelling and facial paralysis. After four weeks of treatment, the tumor mass had almost disappeared, as well as the swelling and pain. After six months, recovery was complete. The patient remained in excellent health and became capable of fatherhood, which had not been the case before the Gerson therapy. His case can be identified as No. 35 in *A Cancer Therapy*. As of August 8, 1957, he was still in excellent health.

The third patient presented was a woman who had had an extensive, infiltrating abdominal cancer. A colostomy had been performed, but her life expectation was put by the surgeon at from six months to two years. Her daughter took her to Gerson, and improvement was almost immediate. After five weeks of treatment, Xrays showed the tumor almost gone. The patient was exhibited before medical students by her family physician as cured; two noted specialists could find no evidence of the original cancer.

A fourth presentation was a woman who had had an extensive lymphatic sarcoma with tumors throughout the abdomen and glands over her neck, axilla, groin and so on. An operation, followed by fifteen Xray treatments, had failed to help her; the patient lost 30 pounds and became too weak to work. After two years of the Gerson therapy, the physician who had originally diagnosed her condition stated that there were no signs of any previous malignancy.

Doctor Gerson testified that her case was interesting from another aspect: After a year under his care, her ovaries were destroyed. Ovarian substances were administered, whereupon her tumors recurred immediately. Iodine was then prescribed, and the tumors disappeared permanently. Dr. Gerson then incorporated iodine into all his treatments because it apparently counteracts the neoplastic effects of hormones.

The next case, too, had experienced recurrence of the tumor after ovarian substances had been administered and relief of the tumorous condition upon the administration of iodine. This woman had experienced the orthodox treatment. In 1940 her breast had been removed; beginning in 1941, a tumor recurring in her neck had been treated by radium and low-voltage Xray at intervals extending over several years. In 1944 her condition was regarded as hopeless, and she then consulted Doctor Gerson. She testified that after only three weeks of treatment her neck tumor began to recede and she was able to resume work. Her tumor disappeared completely and for two years she had been in excellent health.

Dr. George W. Miley, then head of Gotham Hospital, followed to elaborate on Doctor Gerson's therapy. He was familiar with every one of the cases presented, and endorsed the Gerson therapy enthusiastically. In 1942, with Dr. Charles Bailey, the renowned chest and heart surgeon, he had visited Doctor Gerson to investigate his treatment of tuberculosis. He was at first skeptical of Gerson's cancer treatment but, upon observing his cures, became convinced of its value.

Doctor Miley gave this testimony, however, which was to prove almost disastrous for the Hoxsey Clinic:

"A survey* made by Doctor Stanley Reimann of cancer cases in Pennsylvania over a long period of time showed that those who received no treatment lived longer than those who received surgery, radium or Xray. The exceptions were those patients who had received electro-surgery who lived approximately as long as those who received no treatment whatso-ever. The survey also showed that following the use of radium and Xray much more harm than good was done to the average cancer patient. This is a con-clusion which is not generally accepted and is highly controversial among leading cancer workers. It would appear that none of the routine measures employed today to combat cancer are as effective as their proponents would have us believe."

Doctor Miley's testimony was published in two parts which were practically identical. The first part, evi-dently read from a paper, consisted of his verbal testi-mony on the witness stand; the second part consisted of the written statement. The printed version of his verbal testimony contained the footnote denying that Doctor Reimann had made the survey, but the portion which reprinted his written statement did not contain that footnote; this was the only essential difference be-tween them.

In its leaflets, the Hoxsey Clinic reprinted the state-ment which Doctor Miley had attributed to Doctor Reimann. In the government suit against the Hoxsey Clinic in Pittsburgh in October, 1956, Doctor Reimann was subpoenaed as a witness. He testified that he had

---

* At this point, on page 117 of the published hearings, appeared the following footnote: "EDITOR'S NOTE.—A communication from Dr. Stanley Reimann to Senator Pepper states that he made no such survey."

started to collect information on cancer patients from physicians and hospitals in Pennsylvania for the Division of Cancer Control and that this information was intended to be the basis of a real survey. In 1941, however, the Division of Cancer Control was closed and the war halted further compilations. The information collected to that point was forwarded to the State Capitol, but no formal report was ever made.

Here is another cancer mystery. Doctor Miley had been working under Doctor Reimann's supervision at the Gotham Hospital, as he testified before Senator Pepper, and therefore they talked from time to time. In all probability the information gathered was mentioned as strongly indicating that surgery hastened the death of cancer patients. It is also quite possible that the survey was discontinued because the facts would embarrass surgeons and radiologists. At any rate, the government capitalized on its own error and prosecuted the Hoxsey Clinic for false labeling and for publishing in its leaflets that Doctor Reimann's survey had found that surgery, Xray and radium brought death sooner than no treatment whatsoever.

In A Cancer Therapy, which will be filed with the United States Senate when and if it resumes hearings on cancer, Doctor Gerson postulates:

"In my opinion, cancer is not a problem of deficiencies in hormones, vitamins and enzymes. It is not a problem of allergies or infections with a virus or any other known or unknown microorganism. It is not a poisoning through some special intermedial metabolic substance or any other substance coming from an outside, so-called carcinogenic substance. All these can be partial causative agents in man, contributing elements, called secondary infections, etc. Cancer is not a single cellular problem; it is an accumulation of numerous damaging factors combined in deteriorating the whole metabolism after the liver has been progressively impaired in its functions."

Doctor Gerson warns of the perils of irradiation and Xrays, as substantiated in the report in the National Academy of Sciences, "The Biological Effects of Atomic Radiation" (June, 1956). He finds that his treatment cannot benefit those who have received from forty to eighty Xray treatments or sixteen to forty cobalt treatments.

The Gerson therapy requires intensive detoxification with continuous enemas, which must also remove necrotic cancer tissue. Gerson confesses having lost patients in his early years of treatment because he was unaware of the need to remove dead tissue. Autopsies later proved that some of his patients had died not from their cancers but from the serious intoxication caused by the body's attempt to absorb dead cancer tissue.

Another danger Doctor Gerson warns against is the power of vitamins to induce a regrowth of cancer tissue despite improved spirits resulting from stimulated metabolism. He found that the administration of calcium compound to boys and girls with osteosarcoma also showed remarkable results at first, only to be followed by a rapid and incurable regrowth of cancers 10 to 14 days later.

In 1942, Doctor Gerson experienced the tragic loss of twenty-five of thirty-one patients who had been symptom-free for a few months following the Huggins therapy, which is the administration of hormones of the opposite sex. Although patients had felt much better after a few weeks of this therapy, their cancers became worse than ever. This disaster threw Doctor Gerson into such a deep depression that he almost lost the desire to continue working in cancer therapy. The sad-

dest death was that of his "young and hopeful friend,
J. G."*

Every cancer therapy has some unusual feature. Gerson's is unique because it employs no special discovery
or medicament but is based solely on corrective metabolic processes through the foods, vitamins, minerals
and extracts universally available. Doctor Gerson is
himself an excellent example of the value of his diet,
for he has followed it faithfully for over forty years.
Despite his advanced age, he recently flew from New
York to Los Angeles at the request of a patient, re-
turning the following day.

Despite the fact that the Gerson therapy is based
on authentic physiology, discoveries in biochemistry
and nutrition, it has met the usual blackout. The originator is isolated; the medical journals will not publish
his work. His diet, according to the Council on Pharmacy, is said "to make the body highly hypersensitive,
so that ordinary anesthesia might be fatal, a conjecture
that is wholly unfounded and apparently designed to
appeal to the cancer victim already fearful of a surgical operation which might offer the only effective
means for eradication of the disease. . . . There is no
scientific evidence that the dietary intake of food or
other nutritional essentials are of any specific value in
the control of cancer."†

Nevertheless, the evidence Doctor Gerson submitted

---

* John Gunther, Jr., son of the famous author of *Inside Europe, Inside Russia*, etc., who published his son's case history as *Death Be Not
Proud*. This is a full account of his frantic quest for a cancer cure,
undertaken at enormous expense with famous specialists and provides
an excellent insight into orthodox treatment as carried out in our most
celebrated institutions. When Gunther's son was put on the Gerson
therapy, he showed remarkable improvement and a cure seemed on the
way, until the fatal relapse occurred.

---

† As quoted in Doherty, Beka: *Cancer*, New York: Random House,
1949.

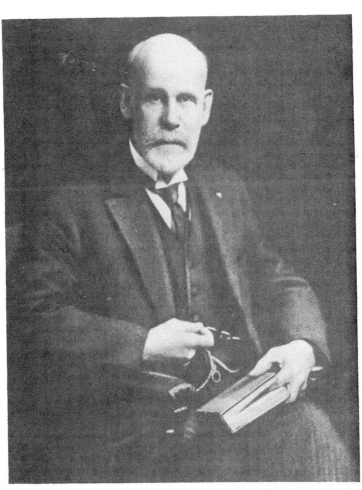

Lucius Duncan Bulkley, M.D.

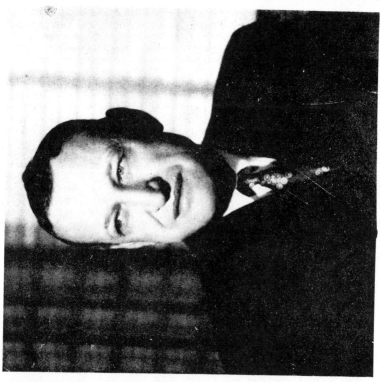

HARRY M. HOXSEY

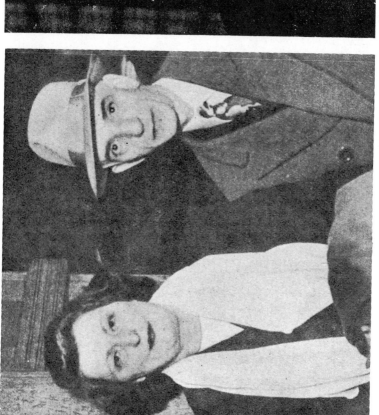

MRS. LILLIAN LAZENBY AND PHILIP DROSNES

to Senator Pepper as extended and elaborated upon ten years later in A *Cancer Therapy,* proves that diet, together with detoxification and the administration of iodine, liver extracts, minerals and so on, brings significant results in cancer treatment. Improvement or cure is claimed for 50 per cent of the patients treated and his claims are substantiated with a preponderance of clinical evidence.

THE REVICI CANCER CONTROL METHOD

One of the most promising approaches to cancer control is based on the researches of Emanuel Revici, M.D., scientific director of the Institute of Applied Biology in New York City. It is indeed encouraging to find an independent cancer physiopathologist who has adhered to the highest ethical and scientific principles, who has not resorted to unwarranted claims or unproved hypotheses, and who has managed to avoid the usual bitter controversies prevailing in cancer treatment.

Because of its purely chemotherapeutic approach, the Institute of Applied Biology has encountered some opposition. But opposition has not been too pronounced because no proprietary nostrum is involved in the procedure and there could be no accusation of advancing a special interest. According to Doctor Revici, the medicaments he prescribes are well known and available to any physician from the usual pharmaceutal sources. The Institute of Applied Biology offers a purely scientific approach to cancer treatment, based solely on biochemical and physiological principles. A unique and most valuable feature of this approach is an explanation of the mechanics of pain, which is applicable in almost every disease besides cancer. It is ex-

plained in a lucid and readily understandable form in
"The Control of Cancer with Lipids,"[37] presented by
Dr. Revici at the Clinical Pathological Conference held
at the Beth David Hospital in New York City on May
9, 1955.

In reviewing the results of surgery and Xray in cancer for the past three decades, Doctor Revici points
out that the rate of cure still remains small and the
cancer death rate continues to rise. Surgery and irradiation have failed to correct malignant processes despite the fact that they are now being used at practically
their maximum efficiency.

Various chemotherapeutic approaches have also been
aimed at a selective destruction of cancer cells without
harming normal tissues, Doctor Revici states. Chemotherapeutic approaches have also failed due to "the
peculiar nature of malignant process." which he sep-
arates into the following stages, as stated in his paper:

"Although generally considered as a unity, the
differences between an early intraepithelial cancer
(cancer-in-situ) and terminal cancer are so great as
to oblige us to recognize that they are of the utmost
importance in the pathogenesis of this complex disease. While the factors responsible for the trans-
formation of cancer from a clinically innocuous cell
disturbance to a lethal disease are usually considered
as secondary characters, our research has emphasized
the roles of these manifestations and the factors which
intervene to bring them about. We have tried to
correlate each of the successive clinical phases in the
evolution of cancer with the intervention of different processes, and thus determine their part in the
complex disease."[38]

Doctor Revici traces the various phases in a developing cancer according to the anatomic level in which it

occurs. This starts from the cell nucleus and eventually affects the cell tissues, organs and organisms. In this last phase, affecting systemic metabolic changes, it ar' rives at the terminal and fatal stage. He presents these changes in the following table:

Anatomical Level	Physiopathological Process	Clinical Phase
Intracellular and Nuclear	Carcinogenesis	Noninvasive
Cellular	Atypical growth	Invasive
Tissular	Local metabolic changes	Painful
Blood and organs	Systemic metabolic changes	Terminal

This interesting delineation simplifies the explanation of the course of cancerous processes from inception until death. In the nucleus of the cell, cancer probably affects the protein fraction of nucleo-protein, Doctor Revici believes, and does not spread if limited to that level. It spreads if the cytoplasm becomes affected, which is followed by the invasion of surrounding cells.

After having penetrated other tissues, one of the principal manifestations of cancer can be pain "caused by chemical changes occurring in the intercellular fluid that bathes the nerve endings," according to the Revici theory. The vascular changes manifested in a small number of cases by hemorrhages or clotting are the next phase, followed by the final phase, radical alteration of systemic metabolism which terminates in death.

That view conflicts with the theory of cancer as a condition limited to cellular growth which must quickly be extirpated or destroyed by surgery or supravolt ir' radiation, often with the attendant sacrifice of adjacent healthy tissue. Doctor Revici states in his paper that he attempts to control the disease by "influencing the dynamic factors involved in the change of cancer from a localized, nonsymptomatic, noninvasive and relatively innocuous nuclear disturbance to a generalized, painful, invading, deadly malignant condition."[38]

Pain in cancer is triggered by the metabolic changes which unbalance the pH* of the intercellular fluid; the farther the pH deviates from the normal, the more intense the pain. Because the deviation could be either acid or alkaline in nature, it led to a "dualistic concept" of pain.

In pursuing his dualistic concept, Doctor Revici detected significant alterations in the lipids present within the painful neoplastic tissues. He was also able to correlate the change in lipid content with both the symptoms and the abnormal metabolism present. He then concluded that some lipids in malignant tumors were quite different from those in healthy tissues and that these abnormal lipids were responsible for the imbalance in cancer between sterols and fatty acids, the two fundamental groups of lipids.

Doctor Revici's theory of cancer therefore embraces the changes occurring all along the organization of the individual from subnuclear entities until the entire organization is involved. He also recognizes two forms of lipid imbalance—a predominance of sterols with a consequent lack of fatty acids and excess fatty acids with a deficiency of sterols. His therapeutic approach seeks to affect the imbalance by introducing chemicals with the same solubility characteristics of the lipids that are lacking. The following clinical result then takes place:

"Pain due to local and/or alkaline changes may

---

* Hydrogen ion concentration; plus 7 denoting alkalosis and minus 7, acidity.

be relieved; the systemic changes may return to normal; vascular changes, especially bleeding, may be
controlled; and finally the atypical growth of cells
may be controlled or arrested. When all these effects are achieved, the malignant tumor can be regarded as having been returned to a phase of non-
invasiveness.

"All of these changes have been observed following adequate lipid treatment. Moreover, in many
cases significant diminution in the size of tumor
masses and even their complete disappearance have
been observed. Theoretically, such objective changes
in the size of malignant neoplasms can be in part
accounted for on the basis of alterations in cellular
lipids, the body apparently having relatively ample
means of defending itself against noninvasive cancer
cells. One indication of this is the observation that
so-called 'cancers-in-situ' have disappeared without
any treatment."[38]

As the originator is careful to point out, the Revici
method is not always successful. Not all patients respond to lipid administration and there has been a continued need for testing various synthetic agents with
lipids to secure one which would appear more active
upon the abnormal process present. The type of lipid
imbalance in each patient must be carefully determined.
Each excess or deficiency of sterols or fatty acids is
manifested by different symptoms and recognized with
different analyses. Therefore the manifestations for
each case of cancer at various moments are distinct.
Frequent urine tests must be employed to check on the
course of treatment and the influence exercised by the
lipids administered.

Revici has also observed the role of lipids in irradiation, hormonal and mustard-gas therapy, and believes

there are distinct physical changes in the molecules of
lipids after the administration of alpha, beta, gamma and
Xrays. He has discovered that experimental animals
will die after continued irradiation when the amount
of abnormal acids created internally reaches a critical
point. That would seem to substantiate the belief that
irradiation treatment can be harmful.

Doctor Revici further contends that the same changes
in fatty acid composition following excessive irradiation occur after the shock caused by burns, injuries or
the removal of the adrenals.

These observations may also clarify other points in
cancer notably, why surgery is sometimes followed by
remission of tumors. This could be caused by changes
in lipids as related to the shock caused by surgery,
when the shock is beneficial and stimulates the body's
resistance factors.

With continuing research, improvements in the Revici method of lipid and lipidlike agents have been
claimed to bring alleviation of cancer in a significant
number of cases. A promise is held out for better and
better results as greater knowledge and improved techniques are acquired. Doctor Revici stresses the early
initiation of treatment; the chances of cure diminish
sharply when the disease reaches the systemic stage.
He also maintains that often it would be advantageous
to use his therapy before roentgen therapy, since it is
a far less radical procedure which spares normal tissues
and helps to maintain rather than destroy the defense
mechanism of the patient.

The Revici method is the fruit of over twenty years
of research which started in Rumania and continued
for some years at the Faculty of Medicine in Paris.
Exiled by the war, Revici resumed his work for a short
time in Mexico City. In 1946 he settled in New York

City, where he continues to receive the active support
of prominent laymen and physicians. He was installed
as director of the Cancer Research and Hospital Foundation which recently purchased a 177-bed hospital, the
first to be newly chartered in New York City in over
forty years.

On August 16, 1955, shortly after the hospital was
transferred to the Institute for Applied Biology. A
demonstration of results in treatment was held for physicians and invited guests and 18 cancer patients, selected from a much larger group of cases subjectively
and objectively improved, were presented by the various physicians who had treated them by the Revici
cancer control method. Practically every type of cancer in almost every region of the body was demonstrated to the audience.

Every patient had recovered sufficiently to return to
full and active lives. All had been treated free of charge
except for some portion of the cost of their medicines
and for laboratory fees and Xrays. Those hospitalized
had paid for bed and board, but there had been no
charge to anyone for medical services.

The patients interviewed ranged from 8 to 80 years
of age. The oldest patient had been treated first in 1942
and remained cancer-free until 1955, when he suffered
a recurrence on his nose. In almost every case, there
had been previous surgical or Xray treatment before
lipid administration, although in one case, a woman of
thirty three, lipids were the first and only treatment.
It had been initiated only one month before the demonstration, yet her cancer of the lymph nodes, which had
been certified by a biopsy, had almost completely disappeared.

A man of forty five testified that his right kidney had
been removed in 1952. Xray treatment followed, but

the cancer metastasized to his lungs. Numerous consultations with several cancer specialists had left him
without hope of recovery. In December, 1954, he tried
the Revici treatment. His cancer was arrested immediately and some cancer areas in his lungs decreased. He
regained weight, energy, and the capacity to work at
his profession.

Doctor Revici credited the speedier effects in this
case and in the case of the woman treated for only
one month, who had responded so well, to lipids containing selenium in the molecule.

Thus Revici method appears to be a promising and
interesting approach to cancer control and to constitute the ideal therapy. It is free of shock, pain or danger; it does not mutilate or disfigure the body; it reduces or eliminates the need for narcotics; it improves
the appetite and spirits; and once the cancer is under
control, it is a simple treatment to follow. Hospitalization is often unnecessary.

The patients who appeared for the demonstration
reported most of these advantageous results, and their
testimonials comprise one of the most hopeful developments in cancer treatment in our day. In most instances the cases treated had been considered terminal.
Of those who did not succumb during the first three
months of treatment, one-third continued to survive
and showed significant signs of cancer regression, some
to the extent that it was no longer possible to recognize
any sign of the disease.

WACHTEL'S PITUITARY APPROACH

Another interesting cancer therapy which has run
afoul of strong suppression was originated by Henry
K. Wachtel, M.D., of New York City. He denies the

virus theory of cancer and favors the following concept:

"It seems probable that the development of cancer takes place only in the body which has undergone certain pathological changes in the metabolism. It may be that the cancer is caused by some normally innocuous factors when they have the opportunity to act on the body which has acquired the predisposition to cancer."[39]

To substantiate this theory, Doctor Wachtel cites the wide variation in results of experiments to induce cancer in animals by injecting various carcinogenic agents. Some species will succumb easily but others are very resistent to powerful doses of carcinogens. Doctor Wachtel believes the same variations in susceptibility exist in human beings.

The serious disturbances in body metalolism which he has observed in cancer are manifested by hyperalkalinity, hyperglycemia, changes in fatty substances and destruction of body proteins and muscle substances. Nitrogen equilibrium is also upset; cancer patients can excrete more nitrogen than they ingest. Although there is some obscurity on the point, Dr. Wachtel also believes that enzyme metabolism becomes disturbed in cancer.

Noting the general similarity of these cancer symptoms to pituitary disorders, Doctor Wachtel proceeded from the hypothesis that cancer is linked with the endocrine system. He experimented with an acetone extract prepared from the posterior lobe of the pituitary and found that it inhibited the growth of transplanted tumors in mice, while an acetone extract from the anterior lobe of the pituitary stimulated their growth. As both extracts are lipid substances, Doctor Wachtel's work dovetails to some extent with that of Doctor Revici.

In 1950, Doctor Wachtel patented the process of isolating a crystalline lipid substance from the pituitary of cattle and registered the product under the trade name of "Antineol." Up to 1954, it had been tested on over three hundred cases which manifested both the extreme cachexia typical of advanced cancer and evidence of metastases.

Of those patients who survived at least one month, a number of significant responses were effected. Doctor Wachtel claims that 75 per cent of the survivors exhibited marked improvement and regained sufficient strength to return to their occupations, even in instances when their tumors did not completely disappear. In recurrences after cessation of treatment, renewed administration again brought improvement, indicating a similarity of cancer patients to diabetics, who must be supplied a substance their systems cannot provide.

Antineol is claimed to be nontoxic and to bring alleviation of pain and regression of symptoms after only 5 to 10 injections. It would appear to offer promise in cancer, but powerful opposition has halted its development and has made the substantial endowments needed to manufacture the product impossible to obtain. Antineol is therefore not available now.

Certain powerful interests torpedoed the development of Antineol, according to Doctor Wachtel whose career began in Germany. He became internationally known for physiological research, and after escaping the Hitler regime resumed work in New York City, aided by the late Nicholas Murray Butler of Columbia University. He served from 1941 to 1950 as professor of physiology and director of the Cancer Research Council at Fordham University. But when he began to test his pituitary substance, he was removed from both posts and after an initial grant of $100,000 from the late John J. Raskob was exhausted, no other funds could be secured.

Doctor Wachtel has been quite outspoken in identifying the source of his opposition as an international drug cartel. He accuses the cartel of controlling every phase of cancer research and therapy, including the allocation of grants from private foundations and government appropriations. Doctor Wachtel contends that in order to maintain its drug monopoly, the cartel strangles every independent approach to cancer.

His accusations put the cancer controversies on an entirely different basis. According to him, the scientific merits of a new approach to cancer are completely ignored because of the potential financial losses involved in discontinuing current methods.

CHAPTER 11

Ivy and Krebiozen

I︫ᴛ ɪs fitting that this history of suppressed and denied cancer remedies should conclude with the and most grotesque case of all—the Krebiozen affair. This controversy repeats every feature of every cancer dispute that has been reviewed, but on a far greater and more fantastic scale.

From the fate of Professor Andrew C. Ivy after he espoused Krebiozen, again it is evident how dangerous it can be to become embroiled in cancer controversies. The fear of such disputes among physicians is as great as the fear of the disease itself. A physician once told me that nothing arouses so much bitter enmity and heated arguments among his colleagues, as the subject of cancer. This may be due to the guilty recollections of cancer victims expiring who might have been saved; or of the memories of patients pronounced hopelessly ill who recovered under the treatment of a "quack", or who miraculously lived without further treatment. Possibly these guilt reactions and the remorse over exhausting the money of patients and their relatives in futile cancer treatments, account for some of these psychological manifestations which are expressed in hostility and attack.

These guilty memories may also account for the vicious treatment meted out to those who have dared to criticize prevailing practices in cancer. As recounted, from Richard Guy of the 18th century and his counterparts through history, such as Pattison, Forbes Ross,

Bell, Bulkley, Coffey and Humber, Koch, Glover, Wachtel and Max Gerson of today, this animus was a common experience. Some of these physicians had been highly eminent before departing from the orthodox ranks, yet their fate was inevitably alike; all experienced contumely, intrigue and condemnation. Previous reputation meant nothing.

So has it been with Professor Andrew C. Ivy. Before becoming involved with Krebiozen, his position in medicine was secure and virtually unassailable. He was regarded as a remarkably fine teacher, as a scientist of unimpeachable integrity and as an excellent administrator.

In his distinguished career, Doctor Ivy has written hundreds of medical papers and taken part in more than 1300 medical projects. He also collaborated in the writing of a monumental work on peptic ulcer and devised an improved method of artificial respiration credited with saving many lives both in war and in peace.

In recognition of his ability, during World War II, Doctor Ivy was appointed to set up and organize the Naval Medical Research Institute and to direct it for the first year of its existence. After the war, the American Medical Association (later to become his greatest detractor) recommended Doctor Ivy to represent the Allied governments at the Nuremberg atrocity trials, a post he filled with distinction. He has also served as executive director of the National Advisory Cancer Council (which assists in the allotment of funds for cancer research) and ironically enough, also as a director of the American Cancer Society.

Yet once Ivy became identified with Krebiozen, he was forced through the same familiar gamut of ridicule and disparagement. Suddenly the man whom the AMA had recommended so highly to the Allied governments became a pariah. He was discharged from most of his appointments, temporarily suspended from membership in the Chicago Medical Society and his scientific papers become unacceptable. He still heads the Department of Clinical Science at the University of Illinois, but he no longer serves as vice president. From high eminence, he tumbled headlong into the mire of disgrace. The following dispatch printed in the San Francisco *Examiner* of May 8, 1958, graphically illustrates his fall:

EX-CANCER EXPERT AT HEARING HERE

"It took Dr. Andrew C. Ivy just one hour yesterday to reveal why he was once one of the Nation's most highly respected medical researchers and why today his advocacy of certain cancer drugs has brought criticism from his colleagues.

"The man who has stubbornly advocated what most experts regard as a phony anti-cancer drug called Krebiozen . . . (and which) the American Medical Association test proved to the satisfaction of unprejudiced experts was useless. . . . (A test which) Doctor Ivy called 'deliberately falsified and fraudulent—a disgrace to a great and noble profession.'

"Doctor Ivy's strong support of Durovic and Krebiozen and their refusal to reveal how it was manufactured or to release its formula to other researchers brought him nearly complete professional ostracism."

An uninformed reader could hardly suspect from such biased remarks that they defamed one of the most fearless, honest and capable men in American medicine. The reporter's accuracy can also be guaged from this paragraph:

"The legislative committee called Dr. Raymond Kaiser of the National Cancer Institute in Bethesda, Maryland, from the audience to ask whether Krebiozen could have been tested there. Dr. Kaiser said it could have been but 'there was never such a request.' "

Actually, as has been recounted, Kaiser was called back to refute my statement that an independent would not be allowed to direct or witness the investigation of his own remedy. When reminded that no investigation had been carried out in the presence of an originator of a cancer remedy, he had said it was because they had "never been asked."

Actually the National Research Council had evaluated Krebiozen on the basis of the very AMA report which the Doctor Ivy had called "deliberately falsified and fraudulent—a disgrace to a great and noble profession," as quoted by the reporter himself.

This reporter's bias was also glaring concerning Doctor Ivy's account of his visit to Hoxsey's clinic, which read:

"Doctor Ivy then backed up the cancer treatment claims of the notorius Harry M. Hoxsey of Dallas, generally regarded by the medical profession as the biggest and most dangerous quack of them all.

"He said he had visited Hoxsey's clinic and had found in the chemical pout-pourri the latter advertised as a cancer cure, at least one and perhaps two ingredients which might be effective against malignant tumors.

"Furthermore, he added, he saw two or three patients whose cancers had disappeared, apparently as a result of the Hoxsey treatment."

Actually Doctor Ivy had been very cautious and his appraisal could not in any way be construed as an endorsement. He had said only that potassium iodide

probably accounted for the Hoxsey remedy's action
in external cancers and that he believed it deserved
some scientific study, although he was dubious about
its value in internal cancers. Yet his cautious and
highly impartial testimony was distorted to give the
impression of an endorsement of Hoxsey, which could
only result in smearing both with the same brush.

The trick of repeating old accusations without bothering to mention the accuser's reply and refutation, is
of course old stuff in smear tactics. As to the alleged
refusal "to reveal how it (Krebiozen) was manufactured or to release its formula to other researchers
(which) brought him nearly complete professional
ostracism," Doctor Ivy had testified very thoroughly
and emphatically on that point.

The chemical nature of Krebiozen had been disclosed
to the best of their knowledge he had testified, but
their knowledge was admittedly incomplete as it was
uncertain whether Krebiozen was a polysaccharide or
a steroid. But, as Doctor Ivy reminded the committee,
such uncertainty was not unusual in biochemistry. In-
sulin, he said, had not been identified exactly until 25
years after the discovery of its clinical value.

It is a travesty that such honest and forthright testimony should be so unfairly distorted. It is also somewhat ludicrous to realize how incompetent this particular reporter was to comment on Doctor Ivy's testimony
for he failed singularly to appreciate the man's remarkable knowledge, his courage and his complete freedom
from bias and prejudice.

His very willingness to acknowledge visiting so controversial, and this writer's estimation, unworthy a
figure as Hoxsey, is in itself a tribute to Ivy's courage
and fairness. He is completely the scientist, untram-
meled by ulterior considerations. His testimony that

even folklore remedies deserve investigation is typical of his open mindedness. In that respect, Ivy cited the effectiveness of bread mold applied to wounds and infections, known as far back as 500 A. D. Today the value of that treatment is recognized as due to a crude form of penicillin which forms on the bread mold.

As for the proposed legislation to set up a commission, Ivy declared: "Whenever you have a totalitarian committee making lists of what is good and what is bad in medical treatment, history shows it is subject to corruption."

Subsequent events also indicate that the very committee which recorded this testimony, was corrupted and the hearings were as "rigged" as the *Examiner's* story about Ivy was distorted. For the very next day, after Doctor Ivy had left San Francisco and could not be reached for comment, the two chemists, Furst of Stanford University and Kirk of the University of California, were put on the stand. Each testified that without the knowledge of the other, they had completed wholly independent and separate assays of Krebiozen and had come to identical conclusions—that it was indistinguishable from mineral oil.

Their statements were widely publicized. When Doctor Ivy was finally reached and informed of this testimony, his fighting blood boiled. In a notarized statement of June 20, 1958 mailed to the members of the committee, he pointed out numerous errors and falsifications in the testimony of the chemists. He demanded that the committee reexamine them and offered to waive the customary immunity protecting a witness testifying before a legislative committee and to present his proof before a grand jury. To date, this offer has not been accepted.

The history of the Krebiozen affair is replete with such episodes of skulduggery and falsification. The drug itself has never been licensed for sale, despite demonstrations of its clinical value and proof of non-toxicity. Naturally, revenues from sales would finance continued research and the development of manufacturing processes which would make it cheaper to produce and more effective. Through a strategem, however, Krebiozen has been classified as a serum. This puts it under the authority of the U. S. Public Health Service. There is no time limitation for passing on the admissibility of serums in interstate commerce and a manufacturing license can consequently be held up indefinitely. Had Krebiozen been classified as a hormone or as a drug proved to be non-toxic, the Food and Drug Administration would have been obliged to license it without delay.

In order to understand the complete ramifications of the Krebiozen affair, it is necessary to review its unfoldment. It is the epitome of all the cancer controversies, but it is also more than that for it is a fight for freedom of research in which the very scientific prestige and future intellectual achievements of the nation are at stake. For if Doctor Ivy is finally frustrated and his claims never fairly evaluated, it means that it is useless for any independent thinker to ever engage in any research unless he first secures the sanction of the bureaucrats who can dominate research projects.

Krebiozen now represents the only independent cancer approach being sponsored by a man of scientific eminence, and the only therapy with some chance to succeed. Hoxsey and Koch have been virtually eliminated; Gerson is old and alone; the other therapies mentioned at the San Francisco hearings are of little importance.

The Krebiozen controversy also has some unique and interesting features, not represented in any other cancer dispute. When the disagreement arose, for once the two opposing factions were more evenly matched in influence and resources. For once, a cancer controversy was fairly reported, in Chicago at least, and the public was informed through the press, over the radio and on television.

The fact that Chicago was the scene of the dispute is also extremely important because it is the headquarters of the American Medical Association. As a result, the "top brass" jumped into the melee instead of delegating matters to some local medical society. When the mess was eventually subjected to an investigation by the Illinois General Assembly, these AMA leaders were forced to reveal their hand and some of their highly questionable practices were exposed.

Another singular feature in this cancer controversy, not true in any other, is that the principal figure involved is not the original discoverer of the remedy in dispute. In championing Krebiozen the discovery of an unknown and obscure foreign-born scientist, Dr. Stevan Durovic, Doctor Ivy has risked his scientific standing and the honors of his distinguished career. This fact alone, amply testifies to his courage and independence.

The Krebiozen story begins in the 1930's in Yugoslavia where Stevan Durovic taught biochemistry and speculated upon the physiological factors which can provide an immunity to disease. When the war came, he was trapped in the Nazi invasion of Italy. Released through the intervention of the late Pope Pius XII, he made his way to Argentina. There he was joined by his brother Marco, a lawyer and former munitions

manufacturer who managed to retain some of his fortune.

In Argentina, backed by his brother, Stevan Durovic continued his researches as director of the Duga
Laboratories and developed the product which eventually became known as Krebiozen. The Durovics' entire fortune, estimated at $1,300,000 ultimately has
become invested in the product.

When clinical trials on dogs with spontaneous (naturally occurring) forms of cancer proved encouraging,
it was decided to attempt clinical trials in the United
States to secure recognition here. Dr. Stevan Durovic
then came to Chicago in 1949 and enlisted the interest of Dr. Roscoe Miller, dean of the medical school
of Northwestern University. Impressed, Doctor Miller
then telephoned Dr. Andrew C. Ivy and asked him
if he would be willing to investigate Durovic's product.
He was and shortly afterward Doctor Durovic was
brought to see Ivy by Messrs. Moore and Brainard
who were later to become somewhat lurid and sensational figures in the Krebiozen affair.

As history shows, Ivy was quick to grasp the significance of Durovic's hypothesis, which he stated as
follows:

"Every living cell contains a regulator of its prolif-
erative activity which is also influenced by the surrounding environment. This regulator is called 'Krebiozen'—a compound of two Greek words, meaning
that which regulates normal growth as it occurs in repair or response to injury. It controls the permeability
of the cell or the enzyme systems of the cell, so that
in its absence or deficiency anaerobic oxidation and
acidity of the cells is increased and uncontrolled growth
occurs.

"It was further hypothesized that 'Krebiozen' is present especially in the reticuloendothelial cells, which, as is well known, react to various stimuli. When these cells are properly stimulated, 'Krebiozen,' which is not present in the blood (except perhaps in small amounts), under normal conditions, is released and can be extracted from the blood plasma.

"Finally, Doctor Durovic hypothesized that if 'Krebiozen' is supplied, the cells in early stages of malignancy will be normalized and those in advanced states of malignancy will be killed or damaged and removed by phagocytosis [ingestion by the cells].

"The chemical analysis indicates that Krebiozen may belong chemically to the polysaccharides or steroids and related substances which are known to possess specific biological activity in many instances, a suggestion which is amplified by the presence of sulphur.

"Biologically there is much evidence that Krebiozen is a hormone which acts to restrain the unregulated growth of body cells. Observations suggest that it is normally present in every living cell, especially in the reticuloendothelial cells, whose function is to defend the body against foreign substances, bacteria and parasites, and to promote the repair of body tissue."[40]

Contrary to the charges made by detractors, the method of preparing Krebiozen, has been openly revealed, although for purely commercial reasons the mechanics and the equipment devised to extract the substance have not been disclosed. Krebiozen is made by injecting into horses an extract of Actinomyces which is secured from a noncancerous tumor known as "lumpy jaw" in cattle. The extract stimulates the reticuloendothelial cells to secrete into the horse's blood stream a specific "anti-growth hormone". The blood is later withdrawn from the horse and is allowed to clot; then the serum is extracted with an organic solvent which removes the Krebiozen together with fatty substances. The solvent and fatty substances are then removed from the mixture, leaving Krebiozen.

So there is nothing secret about the process except the equipment used, the nature of the solvent and other justifiable commercially and technically confidential data. Inasmuch as the production of Krebiozen had been financed by purely private and personal funds, such secrecy was entirely within reason and universally practiced to guard valuable commercial processes, at least until a patent has been obtained.

Long before Stevan Durovic ever visited the United States and Ivy, unknown to him, a grotesque pattern of obstruction was being woven. Unknown to him, some knowledge of his work had already preceded him through one Senor Humberto Loretani, a part time sec-retary employed by both the Duga Laboratories and a construction firm developing a real estate project.

In 1946, the construction firm sent Loretani to buy pumps from the Bell & Gossett Company, located near Chicago. The order was placed with Edward Moore, vice president of the firm who also had some interesting connections in the medical profession. Loretani's or-der was huge; it is not hard to guess what happened. Probably there was a round of entertainment and the partaking of wine. Loretani's tongue may have loos-ened until he babbled about the highly secret work going on in the Duga Laboratories. His listeners could have dropped a hint that further details would be welcome.

When Dr. Stevan Durovic deplaned at Chicago's Midway Airport in 1949 with $190,000 in cash and 200 ampoules of Krebiozen, he was surprised to be met and welcomed by two men. One was Ed Moore seller of water pumps and the other his friend Ken

Brainard. Unable to speak English, Durovic accepted their assistance. As mentioned, they later took him to Dr. Ivy; they also kept him entertained and helped him to buy a home in the suburbs.

After Ivy had begun testing Krebiozen, Moore and Brainard began to show their hand and dropped a hint to Stevan Durovic that they considered themselves en-titled to the commercial rights to Krebiozen. Although his English was awkward, in his forthright fashion Doctor Durovic immediately put them straight.

The drug was still in the experimental stage, he told Moore and Brainard, and no clinical results had as yet been demonstrated. Moreover, as scientific director of the Duga Laboratories, he had no authority what-soever to discuss commercial or financial matters per-taining to the drug. But the two men insisted on pressing their claim and their persistance became in-creasingly annoying.

"Leave me quiet," the doctor begged them in his quaint language. Then they threatened to take up the matter with Doctor Ivy. Horrified, Durovic or-dered them to "leave him quiet," too. Somewhat crassly, the two men mentioned how much they had done to help Durovic establish his connections here and the time and trouble they had expended in his be-half. Durovic immediately offered them some money in payment; it was haughtily refused. Moore and Brainard were after much more—the distribution rights to Krebiozen.

About that time, Dr. J. J. Moore, eminent as a path-ologist and also as treasurer of the AMA, began to manifest interest in Krebiozen. Reputedly, he had ob-served some pathological evidence of its effectiveness; possibly he might have learned about Krebiozen through his acquaintance, Ed Moore. At any rate, Doctor

Moore phoned the discoverer of Krebiozen and politely offered him the clinical facilities at the various hospitals he served as pathologist. Unaware of his caller's power and influence, Durovic simply replied that Professor Ivy was conducting all the necessary tests for the time being. He did not return Doctor Moore's phone call.

The Chicago newspapers got wind of the cancer tests and began badgering Ivy for news. He refused to comment, but as there was a need to broaden the clinical study of Krebiozen, he planned a meeting to which he invited prospective contributors to support more research, various cancer specialists and science writers on four Chicago newspapers. At his request, the latter had been "killing" sensational stories about Krebiozen. At the meeting, Ivy planned to give them the truth.

That was simply that a promising drug deserved further study in the treatment of cancer. There was another reason for calling the meeting—the imminent expiration of the residency permits for the Durovics. Their necessary presence in studies of Krebiozen would therefore provide grounds for extending their permits. (They have since become citizens of the United States).

A brochure[40], was released to physicians only on March 26, 1951. That day became "K" Day, for it marks the day that Krebiozen ceased to be a scientific project and developed into a heated controversy and a public scandal.

The invitation to convene at the Drake Hotel on "K" Day, read: "Up to January 1, 1951, 22 patients have been observed long enough for us to believe that a preliminary report of our observations to a limited group of physicians and a group of lay persons who have been connected in some way with our study or who are particularly interested in cancer is appropriate and warranted. It is my opinion that the substance merits a thorough clinical study and evaluation since I believe it shows much promise in the management of the cancer patient.

"A. C. Ivy"

Among those allegedly invited, although Dr. Ivy de-nies it, were the mayor, Governor Adlai Stevenson, Senators Douglas, Dirkson and McMahon (whose last days in the throes of cancer were to be dramatically alleviated by Krebiozen several years later), District Attorney Boyle, the Argentine consul, Commodore Albert Barreira of Argentine, J. J. Lilly of the pharm-aceutical firm, Morris Goldblatt of the Goldblatt Can-cer Foundation, David Rockefeller, Paul Hoffman and Charles F. Kettering.

The official press release read much like Ivy's in-vitation but unknown to him, another unauthorized and wildly extravagant press release had also been cir-culated. It was the work of a press relations man Doctor Durovic believes had been engaged by the "wel-coming committee" of Moore and Brainard. An ex-cerpt from this sensational release reads:

"The battle of medical science to find a cure for cancer achieved realization today, according to the announcement of the discovery by Dr. Stevan Dur-ovic . . . . A number of patients who have been cured of this dread disease were present and observed today at a meeting of leading cancer authorities held in the Drake Hotel . . . Krebiozen is no longer a dream. Cancer need no longer signify certain and inevitable death . . . the dread disease has been gen-etically explained today and its successful cure has been realized."

According to Herbert Bailey,[41] the official chronicler of the Krebiozen affair, the author of that sensational

bit of ballyhoo was grieving his wife's death from cancer which clouded his judgment in his fervent hope for
a cure. It is possible, however, that he had been deliberately incited to write a lurid release to embarrass
the Durovics. In this connection, it may be significant
that he immediately disappeared from the Chicago
scene.

But the damage was done. Quick and sensational
developments followed. Moore and Brainard immediately put a price of $2,500,000 on their claim to Kre-
biozen's distribution rights. The Durovics summarily
rejected their claim. Shortly thereafter, there was an
unexpected phone call from Loretani, Doctor Durovic's former part-time secretary, who had flown from
Buenos Aires to demand an urgent conference.

Loretani warned the Durovics that if distribution
rights were not granted Moore and Brainard, there
would be ominous consequences. The Durovics refused
to be intimidated. Whereupon Loretani declared that
if they persisted in their stubborness, all the powerful
influences of a mighty organization (and he could have
meant only the AMA) would forever damn Krebiozen
as a quack remedy and its sponsors as charlatans. This
threat failed, too.

Shortly afterwards, Doctors J. J. Moore and Paul
Wermer accompanied by an interpreter, called upon
the Durovics. They, too suggested that Moore and
Brainard be delegated to distribute Krebiozen. Their
suggestion was rejected. When it began to assume the
nature of a demand, Marco Durovic ordered them out
of the office.

The opposition then began to concentrate its pressure on Ivy—for, after all, it was only his reputation
for scientific honesty which gave substance to Krebiozen. Various callers at his office dolefully predicted

that unless he renounced the drug, all his professional honors, titles and prestige would be lost. One of Ivy's friends put these predictions into a long and remark- ably frank letter that comprises one of the most inter- esting exhibits in the history of medical controversy. The author of the letter had himself experienced a punishing reprisal. After testifying at a Congressional hearing against the use of bread softeners, he had been discharged as director of research for a national baking organization.

His letter informed Ivy that Dr. Paul Wermer was gathering clinical data on Krebiozen which would be published in the AMA *Journal* without consulting him. That advance information was borne out very accurately. The author also forecast, with equal ac- curacy, that:

1. A great furor in the newspapers would follow publication of the AMA reports, censoring Ivy for raising false hopes of a cancer cure.

2. Ivy would be suspended by the Chicago Medical Society. (At the voting by the society which decided to suspend Ivy, the ballots were cast *before* hearing his defense).

3. Ivy's expulsion from the National Cancer Com- mittee, from the AMA Council of Physical Medicine and Rehabilitation and from his post at the University of Illinois. (He was relieved of his duties as vice-presi- dent but did retain his post as Distinguished Professor of Physiology and Head of the Department of Clinical Science.)

"You have worshipped the God of research for many years," Ivy's friend wrote, "but have you stopped to think that after an expose of Krebiozen appears, you will no longer have an opportunity to do research in any reputable institution anywhere?"

He then suggested this course:

"At the very earliest moment, you must have in the hands of the AMA—before their report is set in type —a letter which you will ask them to publish at once, and that letter should be a short one and you can explain briefly that extenuating circumstances led you to report on Krebiozen at the Drake Hotel. You can point out the initial reports given you seemed to indicate that the property had some useful necessity, enough to justify further study, but you must say that since that time critical examination of records forces you to the conclusion that these original hopes have not been realized, and that Krebiozen has no value in the treatment of cancer. Get the statement in a letter that Krebiozen has no value in the treatment of cancer, and you can make any other explanatory statements that you wish. You can even point with pride to the fact that you have never asserted that Krebiozen is a cure for cancer."[41]

For Doctor Ivy to accede would have meant the stifling of every instinct for independence and for free inquiry, and his every feeling of self-respect. To recant would have meant abandoning every principle for which he had fought all through his long and honorable career. That was impossible; Ivy refused to become intimidated by the ominous warnings. His fall from grace followed inevitably.

But the Ivys are few and far between. Many physicians who had once acknowledged that they had secured good results with Krebiozen succumbed to the pressure, and begged Doctor Ivy never to disclose their identities lest professional reprisals be inflicted upon them for endorsing Krebiozen.

On October 27, 1951, as predicted the *Journal of the AMA* published the status report on Krebiozen compiled by Doctor Wermer. It attested that 98 of 100 patients treated with the remedy had died. As was also predicted by Doctor Ivy's friend, the report was made without consulting or notifying anyone connected with Krebiozen. As for the validity of the "status report," at the Illinois legislature hearing several years later, Doctor Ivy testified:

" . . . that 24 of the 100 cases were falsified; that two favorable case reports were watered down; that in two other cases favorable results reported to us by attending physicians were omitted from the AMA's account of these cases; that AMA files contained no more than 20 words on some cases, in one instance the report having been obtained over the telephone; that 40 of the non-falsified cases were so close to death that they lived long enough to receive only two doses of Krebiozen, and that 33 were so close to death that they received only four doses. Obviously, the official Status 100-case Report of the AMA is not a research report at all. It was and is only a 'smear report.' "[41]

The extent of falsification can be gleaned from the fact that on March 15, 1954, 10 patients who had been certified in the AMA report as dead or dying, attested in a letter to the chairman of the Krebiozen Investigating Committee that they were still alive and well.

At the Illinois hearings later, the key conspirators against Krebiozen were cleverly exposed by Commodore Alfred Barreira, once of Peron's air force who proved himself an amazingly clever ally of the Durovics. Deciding to investigate for himself, he called at AMA headquarters and asked Doctor Wermer for information. The man who had reported the drug as worthless, nevertheless said he knew little about it and told him to see Dr. J. J. Moore. Barreira was on his guard at once, when he was ushered in.

Generously promoted to Admiral by the genial Moore, the Commodore then used one of the oldest of all dodges to ingratiate himself. Professing himself hostile to the Durovics because of mistreatment, he claimed having incriminating papers which could embarrass the Durovics and force them to relinquish control of Krebiozen. This dodge worked beautifully and Barreira became an insider. He testified later that when he mentioned how much money Krebiozen was worth, Doctor Moore replied with relish: "We are all interested in money and we have to meet together in order to find the way to obtain it, lots of it, and soon."

Continuing to pretend he had damaging papers, the Commodore boldly pressed for a written agreement to guarantee his share of Krebiozen profits after the Durovics were forced to their knees. According to his testimony, Doctor Moore then referred him to Ed Moore since his position in the AMA did not permit his signing any commercial agreements.

When asked how the Durovics would be destroyed if they refused to yield, Moore replied, according to Barreira's testimony: "If the Durovics have money we will prolong the fight until they spend all their money. When they are financially exhausted they will have no other choice but to sell their rights and we have a buyer ready for that time."

Here again appears that oft-recurring incident in cancer controversies—the plot to seize control of a remedy.

Another dramatic episode in the Krebiozen affair was the firing of Dr. George D. Stoddard as president of the University of Illinois for obstructing Ivy's work by organizing the Cole Committee at the university to investigate Krebiozen. In September 1952, the Cole

Committee prepared a report, but published only two pages of "Conclusions" contradictory to the main body of findings. On the basis of this conflicting report, which members of the Cole Committee had not had the opportunity to read, Stoddard was authorized by the Board of Trustees to investigate Krebiozen further.

The committee then demanded that further Krebiozen treatments be halted pending a complete chemical and biological analysis of the drug. It was demanded that a supply be manufactured under contract with an outside laboratory not obligated to consult the Durovics once they had the manufacturing process. The Durovics agreed tentatively, even though the procedure was high handed, because they were promised their rights would be safeguarded.

The University administrators refused to put this guarantee in writing; Stoddard maintained that their word was sufficient guarantee. With so many outsiders involved, the Durovics saw that their process could never be properly protected and they refused to enter into the agreement. In 1954, the Board of Trustees of the University, headed by Harold "Red" Grange of football fame, voted "no confidence" in Stoddard because of his censurable participation in the Krebiozen affair. His resignation that followed, was accepted.[42]

Later Stoddard published his anti-Krebiozen book, which was held from publication for some time by an injunction secured by the Durovics. This move was unfortunate as it implied an unfair restraint on freedom of speech. The book studiously ignores some of the most salient features of the Krebiozen squabble, particularly Commodore Barreira's startling expose which is reported as follows:

Q. Commodore, you admit then, that you started out with Dr. Moore by telling him lies, is that right?

A. Yes, sir.

Q. And you feel that a lie is justifiable, is that right?

A. Yes, sir. I will explain why, sir.

Q. Well, wait a minute. You feel that a lie is just-ifiable?

A. Justifiable for me; yes sir. And, I will explain why.

Q. You believe the end justified the means.

A. Yes, sir.

The lengthy Krebiozen investigations of 1953 and 1954 brought out a mass of data which was set down in over 6,000 pages. A formidable array of legal talent represented the AMA at the hearings and matters were prolonged by asking the same questions over and over again and other such dodges, until the appropria-tion was exhausted. As is so usual with hearings, a tremendous amount of information was compiled but nothing tangible is accomplished. Not wishing to an-tagonize anyone, the investigating committee white-washed everyone involved in the Krebiozen affair ex-cept Stoddard, who became the "goat."

The opposition to Krebiozen continued unabated. When Ivy attempted to duplicate the Durovic proced-ure for extracting the serum, it again became evident. The owner of a herd of horses used by Ivy found himself harrassed by government inspectors for this or that imaginary infraction. The horse breeder was frankly told that he would be in hot water as long as he cooperated with Ivy,[41] but he refused to be intimi-dated.

Though some serum was extracted and Ivy thus confirmed the Durovic's work, lack of funds prevents maintaining the supply of Krebiozen, now at a very low ebb. Few new patients can be accepted as those under treatment must be maintained first. Another

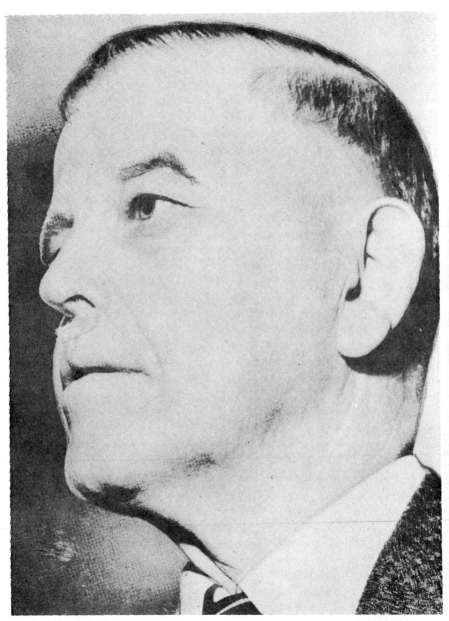

PROFESSOR ANDREW C. IVY

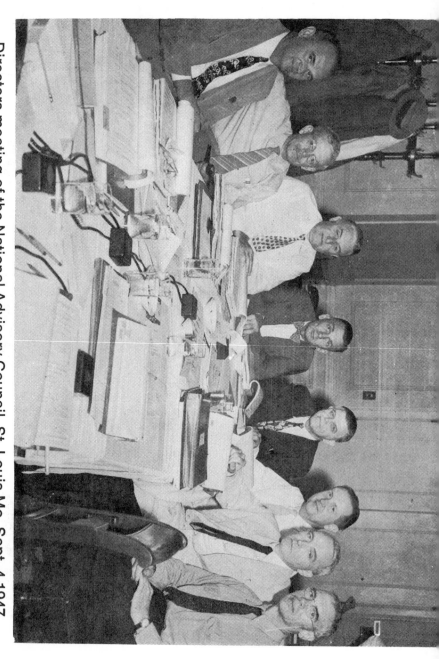

Directors meeting of the National Advisory Council, St. Louis Mo. Sept. 4 1947 with Dr. A. C. Ivy attending. He is fourth from right.

interesting event in the Krebizen controversy was the announcement in September 1957 by the American Cancer Society that it would cooperate in an independent scientific test of Krebiozen. Ivy then instituted a long correspondence with the society, which he once served as a director, seeking to secure some agreement for selecting an independent committee and a fair method of testing.

Ivy favors the "double blind" control method, consisting of two groups of cancer patients being treated, one with the actual drug and the other with a placebo. Neither patient nor doctor would know which had been administered by keeping a secret record accessible only to those directing the experiment.

Doctor Ivy proposed that half of the members of the committee be appointed by the American Cancer Society and the other half by the Krebiozen Foundation, with two additional members to be selected by agreement of both sides. The Society, however, wished to select the entire committee without consulting Ivy. In this manner, the matter of the proposed test was kept in dispute and of course nothing was done. In June 1958, the Sloan-Kettering Institute published a progress report on "natural resistance" to cancer. This report was compiled following much publicized cancer experiments with convicts who volunteered to submit to injections of cancer cells. It was discovered that the healthy subjects readily threw off, and resisted cancer infection but that those with signs of the disease, lacked this protective capacity.

To Doctor Ivy, this meant that the Sloan-Kettering Institute was confirming his conclusions on the immunity provided by the reticuloendothelial system. In a letter of July 22, 1958 to the American Cancer Society, in which he again pressed his request for an investigation of Krebiozen, Doctor Ivy declared:

"The Sloan-Kettering report, as far as it goes, confirms in detail the theory on which Krebiozen was produced, and provides additional evidence showing why our contention that Krebiozen is therapeutically active in some cancer patients should be correct.

" . . . It is gratifying to read in the Sloan-Kettering report their statement that 'There is reason now to believe that natural defenses against cancer exist. It has proved possible, by manipulating and enhancing these defenses, to cure laboratory animals with some type of transplanted cancer.'

"It is further stated in the Sloan-Kettering report, that 'different kinds of cancer may stimulate a common cancer-resistance factor, or that different kinds of cancer have something in common that stimulate bodily resistance.' This agrees with our observations that Krebiozen is of value in the treatment of some patients who have different types of cancer."

In the Sloan-Kettering progress report, mention was made of Zymosan, a drug used to stimulate the resistance to cancer but too toxic for clinical use. Doctor Ivy pointed out the similarity of Zymosan to Krebiozen which, however, had been produced in a nontoxic form.

Doctor Ivy also referred to the statement in the Sloan-Kettering report that "the substance called Cytolipin H in cancer cells which stirs up body resistance in a person without cancer consists of 'two molecules of fat hooked to two moleules of sugar.' " He went on to say:

"In 1956, we reported that the microchemical analysis of Krebiozen indicated that it could be a polysaccharide (a sugar-like substance) and a steroid (a fatty-like substance). Since then, further studies indicate that Krebiozen is 'most probably a polyhydroxycarboxylic acid or acids with some evidence of esterification.' That is, polysaccharide joined to or mixed with a fatty substance.

"The Sloan-Kettering report in summary states: 'If the hunches and hopes of the Sloan-Kettering research-ers are fulfilled by further work, then these achieve-ments could signal a major triumph.'

"Whereas the Sloan-Kettering report states that as yet no application of their discoveries can be made for the benefit of cancer patients, we believe we have at hand a practical weapon against cancer which was produced on the basis of the same theory on which they are now working. Furthermore, I believe if the financial resources were available that the production of Krebiozen could be markedly improved. I said in 1951, it may prove to be a key to "the cure" and perhaps the prevention of cancer.

"In view of these considerations I should like to emphasize the great responsibility which now confronts the American Cancer Society. It is and has been my considered and sincere conviction that Krebiozen rep-resents the only presently available fruit of this new understanding of the problem of cancer to which the Sloan-Kettering researchers are contributing so out-standingly.

"Krebiozen has already been withheld unnecessarily for several years from many cancer patients whom it might help, through no fault of our own but by the excuses of pseudo-critics.

"The decision of the American Cancer Society will determine whether Krebiozen will be withheld still longer from use in cancer therapy until other workers slowly and laboriously duplicate our work *in toto*. This decision is a grave responsibility."

On October 24, 1958, some 13 months after they

had signified they would cooperate in an independent test of Krebiozen, the American Cancer Society indicated how it would discharge that "grave responsibility"— they decided not to sponsor any test of Krebiozen. The reasons given were: 1. The plan (of testing) does not provide for the trial to be conducted by an independent group of clinical investigators recognized as being objective and competent by the scientific community at large. 2. The plan was without an opportunity to determine whether other physicians could obtain the same results as Ivy. 3. It provides no clear standard for measuring either the result desired or the defining or measuring of results obtained.

Ivy's claims for the drug are based on the following observations: Following administration of Krebiozen in cancer cases for the most part advanced, some form of amelioration followed in approximately 70 per cent. Decline of swelling resulted in about 70 per cent, tumor decrease in about 50 per cent, narcotic requirements were reduced in 70 per cent and eliminated for a period in 40 per cent. Favorable results occurred equally among those who knew and did not know they were receiving Krebiozen.

However, on November 13, Mefford R. Runyon announced the American Cancer Society was still interested in a test as, "The ACS would like very much to see this krebiozen controversy settled, and if it (the drug) is of value, that it be made available to doctors and the public. But the testing must meet the recognized standards of the scientific community."

In a telephone interview with Doctor Ivy, he told me that he was still "hopeful" of getting Krebiozen tested. I questioned him about the mysterious phrase "the scientific community," which keeps popping up in ACS announcements about Krebiozen. It sounds

like double-talk, I told him. When asked if he be-
longed to "the scientific community," he laughed
heartily.

As a human being, Ivy is as simple and down-to-
earth as they come. When I first met him several
years ago, I commented upon his quarrels with the
mighty powers of medicine and his refusals to become
intimidated. He laughed, saying:

"What do they expect when they tangle with hill
billies? I'm a Missouri hill billy and the Durovics are
Jugo-Slavian hill billies."

According to Bailey,[41] Ivy was a champion boxer
in his youth. As a child, he is reputed to have bucked
with his head against a billy goat attempting to buck
him down with his horns. As an amateur boxer, he
is reputed to have knocked out men outweighing him
by 30 and 40 pounds.

Another ray of hope for Krebiozen has come through
the efforts of Senator Paul Douglas of Illinois. The
National Cancer Institute heeded his request for a
scientific investigation of the drug and called in Ivy
and Durovic for a conference with Dr. John Heller, director of the Institute and Mr. Frank McCulloch representing Senator Douglas. On September 24, 1958
this joint statement was issued:

"It is generally agreed that the evaluation of Krebiozen should be explored further and we are seeking
to develop an agreed procedure that will be acceptable
to the scientific community."

Again that mysterious phrase! In all probability
though, it refers to the ACS, the National Health
Institute, the AMA, and the Sloan-Kettering Institute
—the very bodies which have consistently opposed
Krebiozen.

The controversy about an acceptable investigatory

procedure somehow seems hollow and absurd. A man of Professor Ivy's proven qualifications certainly is a member of "the scientific community." If he was able to set up, organize and direct a huge scientific project for the Navy as he did in 1941; if he can solve intricate problems in medicine and physiology, as he has over and over again; if he is qualified to be head of the department of clinical science at a renowned medical school, he certainly could be entrusted with the clinical investigation of a new cancer remedy.

However, the purported intentions expressed by the American Cancer Society and National Health Institute to investigate Krebiozen, regardless of whether they are ever executed, at least have some encouraging implications. This "open door" definitely implies that the AMA status report condemning Krebiozen as worthless and the testimony of the chemists at the California hearings that the drug was inert, are no longer taken seriously. They therefore should be regarded as having emanated from non-members of "the scientific community."

The battle for Krebiozen is also being pressed by two lay committees, one in New York City and one in Chicago, the latter directed by Mr. John Davis, a prominent business man. At this writing, these committees are securing thousands and thousands of signed petitions demanding a fair and equitable test of Krebiozen. Senator Douglas is active in pressing his request for a test and regardless of the sincerity of the "on again off again," attitude of the American Cancer Society, it is definite proof that Krebiozen is still not a dead issue. Some day, those who may wish to have Krebiozen administered, may be able to get their wish.

CHAPTER 12

The Cancer Community

The reigning powers in cancer wield a powerful and dominating influence in research, therapy, publicity, teaching, fund-gathering and legislation. They are responsible for the current conception of cancer as a deadly, insidious disease which yields only to surgery or irradiation if caught in time and any other treatment as pure quackery. These notions are iterated and reiterated constantly and tirelessly. Dr. George Crile, Jr., writes:

Those responsible for telling the public about cancer have chosen to use the weapon of fear. . . . They have bred in a sensitive public a fear that is approaching hysteria. They have created a new disease, cancer phobia, a contagious disease that spreads from mouth to ear.[43]

This fear puts the surgeons under constant pressure to operate without the slightest delay. That pressure has had a strong influence upon the practice of medicine, which like any other enterprise, is highly responsive to public demands. The booklets distributed by the American Cancer Society, the bigger life insurance companies, the U. S. Public Health Service and similar bodies, constantly disseminate the importance of the early diagnosis and treatment of cancer. If the growth is operable, immediate surgery is advised; otherwise irradiation is recommended.

Surgeons consequently play it safe; even when they are not certain that a growth is malignant, they will advise surgery. "When in doubt, operate," is their guiding principle because it is much safer to remove a growth at once than to risk allowing to develop into a hopeless cancer. By conforming to the established creed of their societies, surgeons are protected from malpractice suits even though a growth may be benign and surgery may actually spread rather than halt, cancer. If the patient succumbs, they can say the cancer was not reported in time. If the growth does not recur because it was not malignant in the first place, surgeons credit themselves with a cure.

Often these cures are of cancers that are relatively harmless. According to Crile,[43] cancer growths obey no rules. Certain types such as thyroid, and, prostrate tumors may remain small, harmless and localized for many years, even a lifetime. Many cancers grow so slowly they can cause little harm. All these types, regardless of duration or extent, are curable by simple operation. Consequently Crile believes that even if a cancer has been present for a long time, it is not the less curable.

Nevertheless it is dangerous for a physician to advocate any approach to cancer not approved by his professional society. Advising against surgery could incur a suit for malpractice if a patient died. In view of the propaganda being spread, it would be almost impossible for any physician to convince a judge or jury that a patient who died without benefit of surgery would have been just as likely or even more likely to die following surgery.

The surgeons have always dominated in the treatment of cancer, although the recent trend toward chemotherapy has somewhat loosened their grip. Dominence is perpetrated through the power of the AMA and its affiliates to determine the standings of hospitals and the members of their staffs. There are of course some surgeons who are highly capable, ethical and independent minded. They will not be intimidated by their professional groups nor will they perform operations demanded by their patients if they do not think them advisable. That takes courage, and on this point Dr. George Crile, Jr., writes:

More of this courage is needed in the profession. Not every surgeon dares to follow his best judgment in the face of popular opinion. The physicians are as afraid of cancer as are their patients—afraid they will miss a diagnosis, afraid they will cause a month of delay. Many of them believe that this month makes little if any difference in the survival of the patient, but they know it might make a great difference in their reputations. It is a brave surgeon who has the courage not to operate when a patient consults him about her breast.[43]

The domination of surgery, as protested by Glover, Koch, Ivy and other independent cancer therapists, has undoubtedly held back for centuries any genuine progress in cancer treatment. Coffey and Humber were so intimidated they refused to accept patients unless they were certified as beyond further hope through surgery or irradiation.

Only recently has the chemotherapeutic approach become somewhat respectable. The change may be sensed in the protest of Dr. Louis Lasagna of Johns Hopkins University who dared to complain against being forced to test anticancer drugs with "last ditch" patients, as published in the New York Times, March 16, 1958.

In the interests of science and the more careful observation of the effects of cancer drugs. Doctor Lasagna suggested that it would be helpful if drugs could be pitted not only against different types of cancer but also against its different stages. Treating only those patients in the last throes does not constitute a fair test he said because a failure in the terminal stage was not proof a drug might not be of benefit in an earlier stage. One can sense something of the staggering dif' ficulties of independents attempting a new approach to treatment from Doctor Lasagna's complaint, because milder cases were always denied them. Their patients died like flies, but did they really have any chance at all, even with an authentic remedy?

Surgeons are the "glamor boys" of medicine, en' shrined in the public mind as the most talented of physicians, glorified for the deftness of their touch and noted for their quick thinking in emergencies. The best surgeons are bold and resourceful. There have also been surgeons of vast learning who have made original contributions to scientific medicine. The late Dr. George Crile, Sr., one of the founders of the American College of Surgeons, made some brilliant contributions to medicine. Many surgeons have decried the futility of cancer in surgery, from Abernethy, the great English surgeon of the 19th century to Charles Mayo of the 20th. Most recently, Dr. Isidor Ravdin of the Uni' versity of Pennsylvania announced that he was aban' doning the surgical approach to cancer in favor of chemotherapy.

Surgery, however, is the ideal treatment for cancer —from the standpoint of the surgeon. He works quickly and commands high fees for his work. The patient who survives one operation may need another and another as the cancer keeps recurring in different areas. With each operation there is hospitalization, more Xrays, laboratory tests, operating room and an' esthesia fees, narcotics, blood transfusions and nursing care. There is therefore a vested interest in surgery.

Functioning at the government level to maintain the *status quo* of cancer as a surgical disease, is the National Cancer Institute. To impress the public that surgery and Xray treatment were the only approved methods and that the Hoxsey treatment was quackery, even the Post Office Department was pressed into service; placards warning the public against Hoxey and reminding everyone that surgery and irradiation were the treatments of choice were displayed throughout the country's post offices. In this fashion, the government became sales agents for the "treatments of choice."

As has been mentioned, independent remedies will not be tested by the National Cancer Institute on patients previously treated by surgery or irradiation, because if the patient survived it could then be contended their cure was due to the delayed effects of previous treatment.

The joker is that patients seek other treatments only after they have been told by surgeons or radiologists that their condition is hopeless. Such patients are usually the only ones available to innovators of a new treatment; the only exceptions being those who refuse surgery or are inoperable. If they are cured or alleviated, critics can contend they never had cancer in the first place. Since the diagnosis of the disease is so difficult and so questionable, there is always room for doubt and dispute.

The need for a reliable cancer test is imperative. Such a test could immediately establish the value of any therapy and do away with the five year remission as a standard of cure. Despite the $60,000,000 yearly spent in cancer research, not a single reliable method of detecting cancer has been discovered, except the Papanicolau test.

Almost as huge as the government's research centers is that of Memorial Hospital's Sloan-Kettering Institute for Cancer Research. It is engaged in manifold studies. According to the institute's progress reports, these include: The role of hormones in the cause and control of cancer after removal of the pituitary or other endocrine glands; natural resistance to cancer (which Doctor Ivy claims confirms his work with Krebiozen); effects of transplanted cancers in men and animals; viruses as a cause of cancer; fluorescent antibodies and environmental factors in the disease. The latter involves such studies as smoking and lung cancer, the effects of alcohol and the threefold incidence of stomach cancer in Iceland over the United States.

The Sloan-Kettering Institute is always trying to discover a reliable cancer test, without success thus far. It also analyzes the chemical components of cancer cells and hopes to be able to induce the ingestion of some counterfeit substance in the cancer cell to kill it and thus cure the disease. This is only opposite to finding beneficial substances which the normal cells need to combat cancer. Also in the Institutes studies, according to its various reports, is the role of enzymes in cancer diagnosis and the improvement of surgical and radiological techniques.

The Institute has been accused at various times of making unwarranted and unjustified claims. Great hope was once promised for Aminopterin because it had cured Walker tumors in laboratory animals; actually, Aminopterin had been on the market for years and was known to be ineffective. The Institute also continues to endorse mustard gas, although it has never proved of much value in cancer.

Reading the Sloan-Kettering progress reports will disclose that there is really no great difference between

the approach of this high and mighty organization and
that of the independents grimly fighting their own way.
Organizations with the most prestige and money, however, are too wily to make any definite and specific
claims; they merely suggest that their findings are
"promising." As quoted by Doctor Ivy in his letter
of July 22, 1958 to the American Cancer Society, this
is a fair sample of the technique of instilling hope without saying anything definite:

"If the hunches and hopes of the Sloan-Kettering
researchers are fulfilled by further work, then these
achievements could signal a major triumph."

The two biggest fund raising groups are the American Cancer Society and the Damon Runyon Fund.
Both work closely with the government agencies, research institutes and foundations which comprise the
cancer community. Their campaigns to raise money
are masterpieces of ballyhoo utilizing every means of
persuasion, advertising and publicity. One stunt was
photographing from a plane the crew of an aircraft
carrier lined up on the deck to spell out: FIGHT
CANCER. During the annual fund raising campaigns,
post office trucks display placards urging the public to
"Fight cancer with a check-up and a check." Rum-
mage sales run by zealous club women and prize fights
are other enterprises put on for the benefit of the fund.
Obituary notices of cancer victims sometimes suggest
that flowers be omitted and their cost be donated to
the American Cancer Society.

When a new cyclotron is installed, the inevitable
photograph and ballyhoo follow. A beautiful model is
shown receiving treatment under the awsome instrument although an emaciated, feeble and impoverished
patient submitting to its powerful rays would be much
more realistic.

The remorseless drive for money is also pressed through payroll deductions. Nor are soldiers and sailors spared take outs from their service pay. The nadir, however, has been reached from the evidence of this Associated Press dispatch publicizing the 1957 fund raising campaign:

MENARD SETS CELL-TO-CELL DRIVE

Chester, Ill. (AP). The prison banking system at Menard state penitentiary goes into high gear during a cell-to-cell canvass for funds to fight cancer (conducted by) the American Cancer Society. Inmates make contributions through the prison bank, signing vouchers for the amount they desire to contribute. Most of the money contained in 1,700 prison bank accounts is sent to convicts by relatives. Other payments may come from government pensions, Social Security or veteran's disability checks.

This relentless collection indirectly conveys to the public that the enemy is a terrible and savage foe. If the money extracted from convicts is acceptable than all is fair in the war against cancer. That theme also may account for the brutality of some forms of treatment. Malignances are gouged out, burned out, baked, gassed and choked, as a savage would annihilate his enemies.

The same warlike tactics have been inflicted on independent cancer therapists. Those who sponsor the "treatments of choice," boldly malign rival forms without bothering to establish the value of their own. No valid studies exist on the results of surgery, Xray or radium treatment. They are just as open to question as any independent approach, and on the same grounds. Exact statistics on any therapy are really impossible because there is no way of standardizing cancer data.

Crile writes:

There is no field of medicine in which statistics are more confusing than in that of cancer, where the problem is often one of definition. Even pathologists may not agree as to whether a tissue is or is not a cancer. Their science is a biologic science and, as such, is not exact. It is the pathologist's task to predict, from the microscopic appearance of a thin slice of dead tissue, what the behavior of living cells will be. . . . Should every cancer, even a harmless microscopic cancer with which a patient might live for a lifetime, be included in the statistics? Or should we count only those cancers which have progressed to the stage of invading tissue, of causing symptoms, of threatening life? The problem is with the concept of the word "cancer" and with the lack of a precise definition.[44]

An apt example of the difference of opinion possible in cancer, can be judged from a current dispute on the validity of Dr. R. McWhirter's surgical technique in cancer of the breast. After 18 years of tabulating the results of radical (complete) breast surgery, Doctor McWhirter of Edinburgh, Scotland concluded that cancer recurrences were not fatal unless malignancies spread to vital organs. He believed that recurrences could be survived if confined to the lymph nodes. Since Xray treatments seems to control local recurrences, Doctor McWhirter abandoned operations that included removal of the lymph nodes, removed the breast only and then rendered post-operative Xray treatment.

The McWhirter operation was tabulated for two five year periods, and a higher proportion of survivors was claimed than that following radical breast surgery. The techniques was widely recognized on McWhirter's grounds that it eliminated the danger of spreading metastases following too extensive operations. It must

be emphasized that McWhirter's statistics gave an interesting comparison between his technique and the
more radical breast surgery and had been carefully
compiled over a long period.

In 1955, the McWhirter results were analyzed by
a proponent of radical breast surgery,[44] based on a study
of 1,882 patients, treated from 1941 to 1947, 786 of
whom were still living in 1952. It was judged that
13 McWhirter patients had "intraductal papillomas"
instead of cancer, and because 220 patients had also
been subjected to ovarian sterilization, both these groups
could not be claimed as successes. In addition, 203
patients had died after the five-year period and 44
more were dying and even more deaths were predicted.
Other criticisms were; lack of histologic proof that
Xray treatment sterilized the lymph nodes; there had
been severe reactions from the supportive Xray treatments in 47 cases, 3 of which had to undergo arm
amputations.

It was concluded that the McWhirter simple mas-
tectomy spreaded cancer after the malignancy was cut
through—the very danger which Doctor McWhirter
believed followed after radical operations. This was
denied by the evaluator (L. V. Ackerman) who contended just the opposite and disputed McWhirter's
"inference" that the dissection of lymph nodes in the
arm would spread cancer.

This dispute between two orthodox schools of surgery displays the usual wide disparity of opinion also
characteristic of squabbles between orthodox and nonof-
ficial approaches. It proves once again that there really
are no established standards for evaluating the results
of any form of treatment and that it may actually be
impossible to establish such standards because it is impossible to classify cancer exactly. As Crile states, it

is therefore a matter of definition and the way things are run in the cancer community, those with the best and most authoritive positions establish their own criteria purely by force of edict. In that fashion they can disqualify any other definition and establish their own as the only true and correct one.

Cancer is Big Business, make no mistake about that. The treatments of choice are far and away the most lucrative. The treatments not in favor are little business, and the physician who turns away from the orthodox approach sacrifices income for the sake of his patients and principles. He often eliminates expenses for narcotics, surgery and Xray, and reduces hospitalization expense. The blackout enveloping the truth about cancer also hides the frightful costs of the treatments of choice. A leading cancer authority once told me that the way cancer patients are mulct before they die is frightful; sums as high as $50,000 have been spent fruitlessly on surgery and irradiation.

The need for reliable figures on the results, as well as the high cost of orthodox treatment is urgent. Such figures would go a long way toward clarifying the picture and lifting the blackout. The monumental researches of Hardin Jones[1] prove there was no significant difference in survival periods, whether or not surgery was accepted and the patient let the disease run its course. Such scientific studies disprove the propaganda for surgery.

The vested interest in cancer is huge and operates through many different divisions. To summarize, there is the propagandistic or fund-raising branch; the government institutions appropriating millions of public funds; wealthy foundations endowed by philanthropists; the division devoted to treatment which supports physicians and hospitals lavishly. To figure the amount of lucre involved is sheer guesswork. On the basis of 500,000 cancer patients always undergoing treatment currently and an average expenditure of $8,000 per patient, the money expended must be staggering.

Add to this the investment in hospitals, irradiation installations, research facilities and pharmaceutical manufacturing, and you may get some inkling of the cancer community's size. Another new development is also adding to its investment. Researches by pharmaceutical firms in the chemotherapy of cancer are now being partially subsidized by the government. The first firm to benefit was E. R. Squibb & Sons who are undertaking a $7,000,000 program "centering on the endocrine system and the use of steroid compounds," which will be partially supported by the government. Other such projects will soon be inaugurated by other firms.

As this work goes to press, there has been a change in the propaganda of the American Cancer Society. No longer is fear the theme; the fear which Dr. George Crile Jr., said was so epidemic. Now optimism is the word. The cure rate is mounting steadily, claims the American Cancer Society in recent press releases. 800,000 cured cancer patients are now living, the society says, and perfections in diagnostic and treatment techniques may soon result in curing one of every two people who contract cancer. No figures are supplied to support these assertions, nor are any particular new developments or techniques stressed.

The change of front, evidenced by this new note of optimism, may indicate the scare campaign is no longer effective. Doctor Crile's informative work, *Cancer and Common Sense,* the most lucid, honest and informative work ever published on the subject for the layman in this author's opinion, may have had something to do with that.

It is also possible that the public is tired of the eulogistic propaganda the medical profession has been circulating about itself. The practice of medicine has become more and more the nature of a profit enterprise; money is the prime goal. The recent publication of Richard Carter's[45] penetrating analysis of the AMA's organizational structure and its highly lucrative activities, should go a long way toward removing the halo physicians have assumed. The publication of such books indicates the world is avid for the true facts and beginning to weary of the high flown phrases which seem to imply so much but actually mean very little.

If someday the final and complete solution of the cancer problem arrives, let us hope the contributions of independent workers will be recognized; that their enterprise, courage and determination in risking their time, their fortunes and their careers, despite the relentless opposition of detractors, will be honored. If Doctor Ivy's contention is true that the Sloan-Kettering Institute has confirmed his findings without acknowledging the fact, then it is also possible that the final solution of the cancer problem may come from an independent worker overcoming bureaucracy, undisturbed by professional pressure and intent only on finding the facts.

POSTSCRIPTS

Both increased anxiety over the mortality and a rising optimism that the final solution of the cancer problem is imminent, are now current. The public is far better informed about cancer and now expect more from research because they have seen the polio epidemic eliminated. There is also a realization that in Europe cancer is not attended by the witch hunting and derogation of independents that has been so prevalent here. There is greater freedom in treatment and research in Europe, therapy is far more advanced and many Americans travel there to secure treatments not available here.

One in four will be struck by cancer according to current statistics, with a shocking rising incidence in the very young. This has brought into existence the Lamplighters, a lay organization of parents of child cancer victims. In the young, death comes quickly because their metabolic processes are so rapid, the cancers spread so much faster.

It is not hard to guess why children are falling victims of cancer. Kids are the biggest consumers of junk foods; the candies, cokes, ice creams, so profitable for greedy vendors to push are gobbled up by youngsters, amply provided with cash by indulgent parents. It is the same junk polio victims devoured so heavily. The conquest of polio has only brought on cancer in its place.

Another cause for cancer in younger victims is brilliantly explained by Ronald Glasser, M.D., in his magnificent book, *The Greatest Battle*[46] which explains the physiology, biochemistry and pathology of cancer so lucidly, it enables the reader to grasp the latest research. According to Dr. Glasser the seed for thousands if not millions of thyroid cancers was planted the end of World War II when industry turned from manufacturing war equipment to Xray machines for physicians. Almost every doctor and dentist acquired one and became entranced with their magic. They turned up the radiation and beamed it toward the chest to dissolve the thymus of children under the false belief that it prevented colds. They radiated the neck to treat tonsils and adenoids, only to damage thyroids. According to a current news report, "the National Cancer Institute is trying to alert an estimated one million Americans believed to have an increased risk of thyroid cancer because of exposure to head or neck Xrays up to 40 years ago." (UPI)

In his lucid explanation of cell physiology and experiments to induce cancer in laboratory animals, Dr. Glasser proves that any quantity of carcinogenetic exposure, no matter how minute, causes cellular changes which eventually could erupt into cancer, even thirty or forty years later. The news release quoted, confirms this.

Taking cognizance of the increased interest in diet and nutrition, the National Cancer Institute has been compiling data on the nutritional factors in cancer. This also complies with the National Cancer Act of 1974, which includes a provision "to collect, analyze and disseminate information respecting nutrition and cancer, useful in the prevention, diagnosis and treatment of cancer." A grant of $6,000,000 to study the nutritional factors in cancer was alloted and a symposium on the subject published.[47]

But these excursions into nutrition will probably conform to the pattern of procedure the reigning powers have usually set to establish "treatments of choice." Their brand of "nutrition of choice" will ignore the findings of scientists not affiliated with food and drug cartels who strongly criticize commercial food processing.

Though these cartels control billions for experiment and research, some independent workers without their grants are well on their way to a final solution of the cancer problem. They cannot be sneered at as visionaries or faddists because they include some Nobel prize winners. The work of Linus Pauling and Ewan Cameron[48] on the oxygenetic properties of Vitamin C, is a significant breakthrough both in the treatment and prevention of cancer. Incidentally, this discovery confirms the work of Koch whose remedy Glyoxylide was designed to restore respiratory functions to cancer cells.

The scientific explanation for the significance of respiratory functions in cancer pathology has come from another Nobel Laureat, Otto Warburg. As long ago as 1967, Professor Warburg published his conclusions on the nature and biochemistry of the cancer cell[49] He contends that the cancer cell is a reversion to the first form of life on this planet, originating four or five billion years ago, before the existence of oxygen in the atmosphere. This form of life existed through fermentation, a much simpler process than oxidation which requires more than thirty additional chemical reactions to complete respiration. According to Professor Warburg:

> Thus when respiration disappears (in the cancer cell), life does *not* disappear, but the *meaning* of life disappears, and what remains are growing machines that destroy the body in which they grow. The cure and prevention of cancer, therefore, depends upon restoring and maintaining the respiratory functions.

In conclusion Professor Warburg asks:

> Why does it happen that in spite of all this so little is done towards the prevention of cancer? The answer has always been (from the cancer establishment) that one does not know what cancer or the prime cause of cancer is, and that one cannot prevent something that is not known.
>
> But nobody today can say that one does not know what cancer and its prime cause is. On the contrary, there is no disease whose prime cause is better known, so that today ignorance is no longer an excuse that one cannot do more about prevention. That the prevention of cancer will come there is no doubt, for man wishes to survive. But how long prevention will be avoided depends on how long the prophets of agnosticism will succeed in inhibiting the application of scientific knowledge in cancer. In the meantime, millions of men must die of cancer unnecessarily.

It is very difficult to believe that the very centers entrusted with research in cancer at such enormous expense are "inhibiting the application of scientific knowledge in cancer" but it is not so difficult to understand once the economics of cancer is grasped.

The treatment of cancer is after all a business which is very lucrative and very expensive for the customer. The goal of most exclusively profit-minded business men is to sell their commodity at the highest price possible in a market where they can eliminate all competition and customers have no choice but their commodity. Such entrepeneurs secure a monopoly by convincing their customers that theirs is the only valid product available and that competitors are frauds whose product is worthless.

A monopoly of any market is a sure source of profit; a captive clientele has no other choice. The sellers can charge any price the market will bear and can evade any responsibility for bad results because they do not and cannot give any guarantees. They eliminate all critics of their products and challenges to their authority. Their business prospers; thousands of new customers constantly replace those that disappear.

The original John D. Rockefeller was no mean hand at spotting the commercial possibilities in any enterprise. As his millions came in, he kept reinvesting in the most profitable businesses. One day when appendectomies were the rage in the medical profession, a surgeon told John D. that everyone should have an appendectomy before the age of sixteen as a preventative. The oil wizard saw the point at once.

"Why, you've got a better thing than Standard Oil," he exclaimed.

But that was before the days of radiation, cobalt treatment, chemotherapy, and the medical insurance and government financed Medicare which elevates every patient to the status of a millionaire.

THE END

REFERENCES

1. Jones, Hardin B.: Demographic consideration of the cancer problem, *Trans. N.Y. Acad. of Science,* Ser. II, 18, 4, 298-333, Feb., 1956.
2. Montague, M.F.A. and Musick, W.J.: A Yankee doctor in England in 1859, *Bull of the Hist. of Med.,* 13, 217-228, Feb., 1943.
3. Farrow, Ruth T.: Odyssey of an American cancer specialist, *Ibid.,* 23, 236-252, May, 1949.
4. Fell, J.W.: *A Treatise on Cancer,* London: John Churchill, 1857.
5. Pattison, John: *Cancer: Its nature and successful and comparatively painless treatment without the usual operation with the knife,* London: H. Turner & Co., 1866.
6. Walshe, Walter Hayle: *The Anatomy, Physiology, Pathology and Treatment of Cancer,* Boston: Ticknor & Co., 1844.
7. Druitt: *Surgeon's Vade Mecum,* 6th Edition.*
8. Prof. McFarlane, University of Glasgow, *Medical Gazette,* June 24, 1838.*
9. Ferguson*†
10. May: *Outline of Pathology.*
11. Ross, F. W. Forbes: *Cancer; Its Genesis and Treatment,* London: Methuen, 1912.
12. Bell, Robert: *Reminiscences of an Old Physician,* London: Murry, 1924.
13. Bell, Robert: *The Treatment of Cancer Without Operation,* London: Dean, 1903.
14. Crile, G.W. Jr.: Hypothyroidism and Thyroid Cancer, *Cancer,* 10, 16, 1119-1137.

---

* Reference as supplied in Pattison, 5.

---

† A noted surgeon and pupil of Abernethy.

15. Bulkley, L.D.: *Cancer and its Non-Surgical Treatment,* New York: William Wood, 1921.
16. Oberling, Charles: *The Riddle of Cancer,* New Haven: The Yale University Press, 1952.
17. Bulkley, L.D.: *Cancer of the Breast,* Philadelphia: F. A. Davis, 1924.
18. Ozias, C.O.: *The Cancer Problem,* Kansas City, Published by the author, 1930.
19. Christian, S.L., and Palmer, R.A.: Apparent recovery from multiple sarcoma, *Amer. Journ. Surgery,* 4, 188-197, Feb., 1928.
20. Naute, Helen Coley, Et Al: A review of the influence of Coley toxins on malignant tumors in man, *Acta Medica Scandinavica, Supplementum,* Stockholm, 1953.
21. Shear, M.J. Chemotherapy of malignant neoplastic diseases, *Journ. of the AMA.* 142, p390, 1950.
22. Coley, W.B.: Some clinical evidence in favor of the extrinsic origin of cancer, *Journ. of Cancer,* 2, 19, July 25, 1926.
23. Coffey, W.B. and Humber, J.D.: Cancer Studies, *Calif. & Western Med.* 44, 160, March, 1936.
24. Glover, T.J. and White, J.E.: *The Treatment of Cancer in Man,* Murdock Foundation, 1940.
25. Loudon, J. and McCormack, J.: Preliminary report on the Glover micro-organism, *Canada Lancet & Pract.* 64, 1, Jan., 1925.
26. Loudon, J., and McCormack, J.: Notes on the isolation of the Glover micro-organism, *Ibid.* 64, 5, May, 1925.
27. Glover, T.J.: Progress in cancer research, *Ibid.* 67, 5, Nov., 1926.
28. Glover, T.J.: Bacteriology of cancer, *Ibid,* 74, 3, March, 1930.
29. Glover, T.J., and Engle, J.L.: *Studies in Malignancy,* New York: Murdock Foundation, 1938.
30. Koch, William F.: A new and successful diagnosis and treatment of cancer, *Medical Record,* 98, 118, 1920.
31. Rahl, Rehwindel and Redley: *The Birth of a Science,* Lowell, Ariz.: Lutheran Research Society, 1957.
32. Koch, William F.: *Cancer and Allied Diseases,* Detroit: Published by the author, 1933.

33. Hoxsey, Harry M.: *You Don't Have to Die,* New York: Milestone Books, 1956.
34. Gregory, John E.: *The Pathogenesis of Cancer,* Pasadena: The Fremont Foundation,Third Ed. 1955.
35. Beard, John: *The Enzyme Treatment of Cancer,* London: Chatto & Windus, 1911.
36. Scott, Cyril: *Victory Over Cancer,* London: True Health, 1957.
37. Gerson, Max. *A Cancer Therapy,* New York: Whittier Press, 1958.
38. Revici, Emanuel: *The Control of Cancer with Lipids,* New York: Institute for Applied Biology, 1955.
39. Wachtel, H.K.: *The Role of the Pituitary in Cancer,* New York: William Frederick Press, 1954.
40. Ivy, Andrew C., Et Al.: Kreboizen *An Agent for Treatment of Malignant Tumors,* Chicago: Krebiozen Research Foundation, 1951.
41. Bailey, Herbert: *A Matter of Life and Death,* New York: Putnam, 1958.
42. Stoddard, George D.: *"Krebiozen,"* The Great Cancer *Mystery,* Boston: The Beacon Press, 1955.
43. Crile, George W., Jr.: *Cancer and CommonSense,* New York: Viking, 1955.
44. Ackerman, L.V.: Evaluation of treatment of cancer of breast at University of Edinburgh (Scotland) under direction of Dr. Robert McWhirter, *Cancer,* 8, 883-887, Sept., 1955.
45. Carter, Richard: *The Doctor Business,* New York: Doubleday, 1958.
46. Glasser, Ronald J. *The Greatest Battle,* New York: Random House, 1976.
47. American Cancer Society and National Cancer Institute, *Symposium on Nutrition in Causation of Cancer, Cancer Research,* Vol. 35, p3231, 1975.
48. Cameron, Ewan and Pauling, Linus, *Supplemental ascorbate in the supportive treatment of cancer.* Proceedings of the National Academy of Sciences, Vol. 73, No. 10, pp3685-3689, Oct. 1976.
49. Warburg, Otto, *The Prime Cause and Prevention of Cancer,* Wurzburg, Germany: Konrad Triltsch, 1967.

INDEX

203